THE UNIVERSITY OF UTAH
Handbooks in Radiology

Chest Radiology

THE UNIVERSITY OF UTAH
HANDBOOKS IN RADIOLOGY SERIES

Series Editors

Anne G. Osborn, M.D.
Director of Neuroradiology and Professor of Radiology, University of Utah School of Medicine, Salt Lake City, Utah

David G. Bragg, M.D.
Professor and Chairman, Department of Radiology, University of Utah School of Medicine, Salt Lake City, Utah

---

Nuclear Medicine
Frederick L. Datz, M.D.

Neuroradiology: Skull and Brain
Anne G. Osborn, M.D., H. Ric Harnsberger, M.D., Wendy R. K. Smoker, M.D.

Skeletal Radiology
B. J. Manaster, M.D.

Neuroradiology: Head and Neck
H. Ric Harnsberger, M.D., Wendy R. K. Smoker, M.D., Anne G. Osborn, M.D.

Ultrasonography
Donald A. Cubberley, M.D., William J. Zwiebel, M.D.

Angiography
Myron M. Wojtowycz, M.D.

Neuroradiology: Spine and Spinal Cord
Wendy R. K. Smoker, M.D., B. J. Manaster, M.D., Anne G. Osborn, M.D., H. Ric Harnsberger, M.D.

THE UNIVERSITY OF UTAH
Handbooks in Radiology

Chest Radiology

Howard Mann, M.D.
Assistant Professor of Radiology
University of Utah School of Medicine
University of Utah Hospital
Salt Lake City, Utah

David G. Bragg, M.D.
Professor and Chairman
Department of Radiology
University of Utah School of Medicine
Salt Lake City, Utah

YEAR BOOK MEDICAL PUBLISHERS, INC.
CHICAGO • LONDON • BOCA RATON

Copyright © 1989 by Year Book Medical Publishers, Inc. All rights reserved. No part of this publication may be reproduced, stored in a retrieval system, or transmitted, in any form or by any means—electronic, mechanical, photocopying, recording, or otherwise—without prior written permission from the publisher. Printed in the United States of America.

1 2 3 4 5 6 7 8 9 0 P R 93 92 91 90 89

Library of Congress Cataloging-in-Publication Data

Mann, Howard.
　Chest radiology.

　(The University of Utah handbooks in radiology)
　Includes bibliographies and index.
　1. Chest—Radiography—Handbooks, manuals, etc.
2. Chest—Diseases—Diagnosis—Handbooks, manuals, etc.
I. Bragg, David G., 1933-　　. II. Title.　III. Title: Chest radiology.　IV. Series. [DNLM: 1. Thoracic Radiography—handbooks.　WF 39 M281h]
RC941.M35　1989　　　617'.5407572　　　88-26163
ISBN 0-8151-5758-4

Sponsoring Editor: James D. Ryan
Associate Managing Editor, Manuscript Services:
　Deborah Thorp
Production Project Manager: Carol A. Reynolds
Proofroom Manager: Shirley E. Taylor

Contributors

David G. Bragg, M.D.
Professor and Chairman
Department of Radiology
University of Utah School of Medicine
Salt Lake City, Utah

Patrick B. Brown, M.D.
Department of Radiology
University of Washington Medical Center
Seattle, Washington

Virgil R. Condon, M.D.
Associate Professor of Radiology
University of Utah School of Medicine
Director of Pediatric Radiology
Primary Children's Medical Center
Salt Lake City, Utah

Howard Mann, M.D.
Assistant Professor of Radiology
University of Utah School of Medicine
University of Utah Hospital
Salt Lake City, Utah

Editor's Introduction and Preface

Chest Radiology, the second text in *The University of Utah Handbooks in Radiology* series, is written as an introduction for the medical student, beginning radiology resident, and non-radiologist clinician interested in chest diseases. The major pulmonary abnormalities have been subdivided into 12 categories, including a miscellaneous section that includes entities not covered in any of the major disease topics. In addition, a category on intensive care radiology has been included to address the unique problems found in the ICU setting, such as the mechanical support systems visible on the portable chest x-ray in that setting.

In each of the categories, the clinical and pathologic conditions have been reviewed in order to place them in the perspective of the radiographic abnormalities. One cannot hope to understand or play a significant role in the diagnosis and posttreatment follow-up of any of these conditions without a clear understanding of the embryologic, clinical, or pathologic basis for each entity. In many cases, the medical or surgical treatment will have a major impact on the radiographic evolution of the disease process, and one should clearly understand the types of treatments utilized and their impact on the chest x-ray.

In the chapter on lung injury, the effects of iatrogenic injury, including drugs, catheters, and radiation, are covered in a summary fashion within each specific section.

Both space and the format of this introductory text preclude any detailed discussion of radiation biology, technical considerations, and procedures such as angiography. Recommended reading and bibliographic references will help direct the reader to a more in-depth coverage of specific entities in each section.

It is hoped that through this introductory text, the reader will gain a greater appreciation for the significant role of chest radiology in the spectrum of pulmonary diseases. For those of you just beginning the study of chest radiology, it is hoped that this handbook will serve as a catalyst for a more in-depth review of the subject, and that for others it will provide an appropriate introduction to and review of this complex set of pulmonary abnormalities.

David G. Bragg, M.D.

Contents

Editor's Introduction and Preface vii

1 / The Newborn Chest 1

    EMBRYOLOGY 2

    PULMONARY CAUSES OF RESPIRATORY DISTRESS 3

        Hyaline Membrane Disease 4

        Transient Tachypnea of the Newborn 6

        Bronchopulmonary Dysplasia 6

        Wilson-Mikity Syndrome (Pulmonary Dysmaturity) 7

        Neonatal Pneumonias 7

        Persistent Fetal Circulation 8

        Infant of a Diabetic Mother 9

        Pulmonary Development Abnormalities 9

    NEONATAL CONGESTIVE HEART FAILURE 18

MEDIASTINAL CAUSES OF NEONATAL RESPIRATORY DISTRESS 19

Anterior Mediastinal Masses 19
Middle Mediastinal Masses 20
Posterior Mediastinal Masses 20

CHEST WALL CAUSES OF NEONATAL RESPIRATORY DISTRESS 21

2 / Pulmonary Infections 23

GENERAL CONSIDERATIONS 23

BACTERIAL PNEUMONIA 24

Gram-Positive Cocci 24
Aerobic Gram-Negative Organisms 26
Anaerobic Bacillary Pneumonia and Aspiration Pneumonia 30

VIRAL PNEUMONIAS 32

Viral Pneumonias in Adults 32
Viral Pneumonias in Immunocompromised Hosts 33

THE ATYPICAL PNEUMONIAS 34

Mycoplasma Pneumonia 34
Psittacosis 35

MYCOBACTERIAL INFECTIONS 37

Tuberculosis 37

PULMONARY DISEASE CAUSED BY NONTUBERCULOUS MYCOBACTERIA *41*

ACTINOMYCOSIS AND NOCARDIASIS *42*

   Actinomycosis *42*

   Nocardiasis *43*

PULMONARY FUNGAL INFECTIONS *43*

   Histoplasmosis *44*

   Coccidioidomycosis *46*

   North American Blastomycosis *48*

   Aspergillosis *49*

   Cryptococcosis *51*

   Phycomycosis *51*

CANDIDIASIS *52*

   Radiography *52*

PROTOZOA *52*

THE IMMUNOSUPPRESSED HOST: A GUIDE TO PREDOMINANT PATHOGENS IN SPECIFIC CLINICAL SITUATIONS *53*

CHEST RADIOGRAPHY AND PATTERN RECOGNITION IN THE IMMUNOCOMPROMISED HOST *53*

3 / **Neoplastic Diseases of the Thorax** *58*

XII *Contents*

    CHEST WALL NEOPLASMS   *58*

        Radiography   *60*

    PLEURAL NEOPLASMS   *60*

        Radiography   *60*

    MEDIASTINUM   *62*

        Radiography   *71*

    PRIMARY LUNG NEOPLASMS   *71*

        Radiography   *79*

    PULMONARY METASTATIC DISEASE   *79*

        Radiography   *83*

4 / Pulmonary Hypertension and Edema   *86*

    PULMONARY HYPERTENSION   *86*

        Definition and Terminology   *86*

        Radiography of Pulmonary Hypertension   *89*

        Diagnostic Approach to Pulmonary Hypertension   *90*

        A Guide to Imaging Procedures in the Evaluation of Pulmonary Hypertension   *93*

    PULMONARY EDEMA   *95*

        Pathophysiology of Pulmonary Edema   *95*

        Sequence of Fluid Accumulation in the Lung   *97*

Radiography of Pulmonary Edema 97

Radiographic Differentiation Between Hydrostatic and Increased-Permeability Pulmonary Edema 99

5 / Pulmonary Thromboembolism 105

ACUTE PULMONARY EMBOLISM 105

Pathophysiology 106

Clinical Diagnosis 107

CHRONIC (PROXIMAL) PULMONARY THROMBOEMBOLISM 116

Pulmonary Tumor Embolism 116

Pulmonary Fat Embolism 117

Pulmonary Septic Embolism 118

6 / The Trachea 121

TRACHEAL DIMENSIONS 121

DIFFUSE TRACHEAL NARROWING 121

Fungal Infections 121

Tuberculosis 123

Wegener's Granulomatosis 123

Relapsing Polychondritis 123

Sarcoidosis 124

Amyloidosis 124

Tracheopathia Osteochondroplastica   *124*

Saber-Sheath Trachea   *124*

Idiopathic Mediastinal Fibrosis   *125*

DIFFUSE TRACHEAL WIDENING   *125*

Mounier-Kühn Syndrome (Tracheobronchomegaly)   *125*

Tracheal Dilatation in Disorders of Connective Tissue   *125*

RADIOGRAPHIC ASSESSMENT OF TRACHEAL MORPHOLOGY   *125*

FLUOROSCOPIC ASSESSMENT OF TRACHEAL DYNAMICS   *126*

7 / Chronic Bronchial Disease   *127*

DEFINITIONS AND PATHOPHYSIOLOGY   *127*

CHRONIC BRONCHITIS   *128*

Radiography   *128*

ASTHMA   *129*

Radiography   *129*

ALLERGIC BRONCHOPULMONARY ASPERGILLOSIS   *130*

BRONCHIECTASIS   *132*

Radiography   *133*

IMMOTILE CILIA SYNDROME   *133*

Contents **XV**

- CYSTIC FIBROSIS *134*
  - Radiography *134*
- BRONCHIOLITIS OBLITERANS *136*
  - Radiography *136*

8 / Emphysema *139*
- DEFINITION *139*
- MORPHOLOGIC CATEGORIES *140*
  - Centrilobular (Centriacinar) Emphysema *140*
  - Panacinar Emphysema *140*
  - Paraseptal Emphysema *141*
  - Irregular Emphysema *141*
- RADIOGRAPHY *141*
  - Lung Hyperinflation *142*
  - Radiolucent Areas With Vascular Attenuation *142*
- PULMONARY HYPERTENSION IN EMPHYSEMA *142*
- PULMONARY EDEMA AND PNEUMONIA IN EMPHYSEMA *143*
- COMPUTED TOMOGRAPHY IN EMPHYSEMA *143*

9 / Occupational Lung Disease *145*
- INORGANIC DUST PNEUMOCONIOSIS *146*

Asbestosis *146*

Asbestos-Related Pleural Disease *147*

Asbestos-Related Parenchymal Abnormalities *151*

Silicosis *152*

Coal Worker's Pneumoconiosis *153*

Berylliosis *154*

HYPERSENSITIVITY PNEUMONITIS *155*

Pathogenesis *155*

Clinical Presentation and Diagnosis *156*

Radiography *156*

10 / Pulmonary Vasculitis *158*

PATHOLOGIC DEFINITIONS *159*

PATHOGENETIC MECHANISMS IN VASCULITIS *160*

CLASSIFICATION OF THE VASCULITIC SYNDROMES *161*

Wegener's Granulomatosis *161*

Allergic Angiitis and Granulomatosis (Churg-Strauss Phenomenon) *164*

Polyarteritis Nodosa *165*

Hypersensitivity Vasculitis *165*

Temporal Arteritis *166*

Takayasu's Arteritis *166*

Contents **XVII**

    Immune Complex Disease and Vasculitis in Other Disorders   *167*

    RADIOLOGIC-PATHOLOGIC CORRELATION   *167*

11 / Lung Injury   *169*

    PENETRATING TRAUMA   *169*

    BLUNT CHEST TRAUMA   *170*

        General Features   *170*
        Chest Wall   *171*
        Pleura   *172*
        Lung Parenchyma   *173*
        Mediastinum   *174*
        Diaphragmatic Rupture   *176*

    RADIATION INJURY   *177*

        Pathology   *177*
        Clinical Course   *178*
        Radiographic Course   *179*

    DRUG INJURY   *180*

    INHALATIONAL INJURIES   *186*

        Noxious Gases and Aerosol Exposure   *186*
        Smoke Inhalation   *187*
        Thermal Injury   *187*

12 / Chronic Infiltrative Lung Disease   *190*

RADIOGRAPHY OF DIFFUSE INFILTRATIVE PULMONARY DISEASE 191

SPECIFIC INFILTRATIVE DISORDERS 193

Usual Interstitial Pneumonia 193

Desquamative Interstitial Pneumonia 194

Pulmonary Lymphoid Hyperplasia 195

Sarcoidosis 196

Primary Pulmonary Histiocytosis 198

Pulmonary Lymphangiomyomatosis 200

Rheumatoid Arthritis 201

Scleroderma (Progressive Systemic Sclerosis) 202

Systemic Lupus Erythematosus 203

Pulmonary Hemosiderosis 203

Pulmonary Eosinophilia 204

Pulmonary Amyloidosis 204

DIAGNOSTIC APPROACH TO DIFFUSE INFILTRATIVE DISEASE AND INTERSTITIAL FIBROSIS 206

PATTERN RECOGNITION AND DESCRIPTION OF RADIOGRAPHIC SHADOWS 206

13 / Chest Radiography in the Intensive Care Unit   *210*

    MOBILE RADIOGRAPHY   *211*

        Exposure Times   *211*

        Patient Positioning   *211*

        Exposure Latitude, Radiographic Contrast, and Kilovolt (Peak)   *211*

    AN APPROACH TO RADIOGRAPHIC INTERPRETATION   *212*

    MODE OF VENTILATION AND LUNG VOLUMES   *212*

    PLACEMENT OF INTRAVASCULAR CATHETERS, TUBES, AND DRAINS   *215*

    BAROTRAUMA   *217*

    EXTRAVASCULAR AND INTRAVASCULAR FLUID STATUS   *218*

    PROGRESSION/REGRESSION OF KNOWN CARDIOPULMONARY DISEASE   *220*

Index   *222*

1

The Newborn Chest

David G. Bragg, M.D.
Patrick Brown, M.D.
Virgil R. Condon, M.D.

KEY CONCEPTS

1. The normal position of the right hemidiaphragm dome is the eighth to ninth posterior rib. Reduced lung volumes should only be seen with hyaline membrane disease and congestive heart failure (CHF).

2. Transient tachypnea of the newborn may resemble CHF and occurs more commonly in newborns delivered by cesarian section.

3. Barotrauma is visible as a coarse, cystic air-bronchogram pattern extending to the periphery of the lung. The pneumothorax of the newborn often is subtle and is usually located anteromedially.

4. The unilateral opaque newborn lung with mediastinal shift is an urgent diagnostic problem with differential considerations including congenital diaphragmatic hernia, congenital lobar emphysema, and cystic adenomatoid malformation.

5. Neonatal CHF is usually caused by obstructive left heart lesions, total anomalous pulmonary venous return with obstruction, volume overload, and high-output states.

Interpretation and evaluation of the newborn chest are among the more challenging tasks in plain-film radiology. The physiologic changes that the neonatal cardiopulmonary system is undergoing further complicate radiologic diagnosis. The properly exposed chest radiograph is a critical determinant in the evaluation of the newborn who is clinically classified as suffering from neonatal respiratory distress. The radiograph must virtually always be obtained on portable equipment and should be well collimated to include only the chest, if possible utilizing rare earth or at least, high-speed screens, and generally exposed within a range of 50 to 60 kilovolt (peak) kV(p). A short exposure time should be cued to maximal inspiration whether mechanical ventilation is utilized or not. The infant should be positioned in a directly anteroposterior (AP) supine projection with the ventilatory tubes and lines removed from a location where they might superimpose the chest on the AP radiograph. A slight caudal tube angulation or elevation of the infant's shoulders will help prevent an apical lordotic projection. The difference between AP supine radiographs at full inspiration and expiration can mimic dramatic physiologic and pathologic abnormalities, so that this possibility should be considered whenever a dramatic technical change is noted between two consecutive studies.

EMBRYOLOGY

The survival of the premature infant is dependent on the maturity of the lungs as well as any associated underlying congenital defects or acquired diseases. The embryologic lung buds initially appear within the first month after conception. Shortly thereafter, these buds form lobar bronchi and then begin their dichotomous branching until the adult lobar anatomy is established at approximately 12 gestational weeks. By 20 to 24 weeks, capillaries begin to envelop the supporting stroma of the lung, and type I and II pneumocytes begin to form, with type II pneumocytes producing surfactant. The lung is capable of independently supporting life by 28 to 30 weeks even though the lung continues to grow with alveolar proliferation until the child is approximately 8 years of age, at which time the alveoli are numerically equivalent to those in the adult lung.

If one assumes that respiratory distress is caused by a number of pulmonary and nonpulmonary abnormalities, one can separate these disorders based on time of presentation, clinical course, and radiographic characteristics. There are extrapulmonary causes of respiratory distress that are related to congenital heart disease, esophageal atresia and fistula, diaphragmatic hernias, neuromuscular disorders, central nervous system depression or injury, mediastinal masses, and chest wall anomalies.

PULMONARY CAUSES OF RESPIRATORY DISTRESS

Radiographs of the newborn chest immediately following birth should be interpreted with caution and conservatism. In intrauterine life, the lungs are filled with fluid, and in the first few moments following delivery, the lung must clear itself of this fluid and achieve adequate expansion. The thymocardiac image is characteristically large and initially may appear as if underlying cardiac disease may be present. Without intubation, the dome of the hemidiaphragms on full inspiration should reach at least the posterior eighth rib. The level of inspiration may be artifactually distorted once the child has been intubated. Catheter positions should be carefully checked to be certain that the umbilical artery catheter is not in a position to compromise the renal arteries or celiac axis. Arterial catheter termination between T-6 and T-9 or L-2 and L-4 is preferred. The umbilical venous catheter should ideally be placed in either the ductus venosus, the hepatic vein, or the right atrium. The most common complications of catheters are thrombosis of the major vessels and resulting bowel, renal, and lower extremity ischemia; less common complications are infection and the subsequent development of aneurysms and perforation. It is estimated that in 3% of all umbilical artery catheterizations some form of complication develops. The endotracheal tube ideally should be in the midthoracic trachea. Significant variation in position of the tube between examinations may occur with changes in the flexion or extension of the infant's neck without actual change in tube position. An orogastric tube should be in the stomach to prevent gastric distention, which acts to mechanically impair left hemidiaphragmatic motion and stimulates the vagus nerve to cause bradycardia.

Hyaline Membrane Disease

Hyaline membrane disease (HMD) is the most common cause of respiratory distress in the premature infant. Predisposing conditions include maternal diabetes, cesarian section delivery, and perinatal asphyxia. The process results from a deficiency of surfactant, with secondary alveolar membrane damage leading to the development of diffuse air-space consolidation producing air bronchograms and low lung volumes. Classic roentgenographic findings are a reticulogranular appearance in the mild to moderate cases, progressing to near complete opacification of the lungs in the more severe cases. Well-defined air bronchograms can be seen extending well into the peripheral lung. HMD begins some hours following birth and usually runs its course within 7 to 10 days. Often, the pattern and course of the disease are complicated by subsequent bronchopulmonary dysplasia, extraventilatory air, congestive heart failure, pulmonary hemorrhage, atelectasis, or patent ductus arteriosis (PDA). Often, PDA develops as a complication in the patient with HMD, occurring in response to multiple factors including hypoxia, prolonged mechanical ventilation, and increased pulmonary vascular resistance, during the first 2 weeks of an infant's life, and evidenced by increasing heart size, inability to wean the infant from ventilatory support, and, occasionally, pulmonary edema. In efforts to ventilate the child, pulmonary interstitial emphysema, pneumomediastinum, and pneumothorax may result from barotrauma secondary to increasing ventilatory pressure requirements.

Pulmonary interstitial emphysema (PIE) is characterized by extraventilatory air within the visceral pleural compartment and interlobular septa. Air may also be found in the pulmonary lymphatics that parallel or occupy the interlobular septa, which may explain some of the clinical behavior of patients with PIE. The presence of air in the pulmonary interstitium decreases compliance and adds a further barrier to gas exchange, creating a vicious cycle of a demand for increased ventilatory pressures yet a greater risk for the development of a pneumothorax. The radiographic features of PIE must be distinguished from those of HMD. They are characterized by a more vivid "air bronchogram" representing interstitial air that has dissected along the bronchovascular sheaths to the pleural surface. Well-defined 1- to 2-mm cysts—which may progress to form sizable pneumatoceles several centimeters in diameter—may also be seen. Pneumomediastinum and pneumopericardium may also be a consequence of barotrauma, even though a pneumothorax is the more commonly observed complication of PIE.

Roentgenographic features of a pneumomediastinum are hyperlucent areas adjacent to the mediastinal contour demarcated by the pleural reflection. The thymus is often elevated, with air extending medially below its inferior border, producing the "spinnaker sail sign." Mediastinal air in the newborn does not extend into the neck but occasionally dissects into the abdomen. Pneumomediastinum must be differentiated from life-threatening pneumopericardium. The reflections of the pericardial sac extend just cranial to the pulmonary outflow tract and caudal to the aortic arch. In the typical pneumopericardium, air extends between the heart and diaphragm and around the lateral borders of the heart, producing a "halo effect."

A pneumothorax in the newborn infant, as viewed in a portable chest radiograph with the patient supine, is often difficult to recognize. Free intrapleural air most often collects in the anterior medial pleural space contiguous with the cardiac border, increasing the sharp margination of the cardiac silhouette. Less frequently, air can be seen in a subpulmonic location, appearing as if the dome of the hemidiaphragm has become more vividly outlined. Anterolateral pneumothoraces are next in frequency, with the least common location for pneumothorax being apical, as one would expect in a radiograph with the patient erect. Cross-table lateral and decubitus radiographs are frequently helpful to exclude or diagnose a pneumomediastinum or pneumothorax.

Transient Tachypnea of the Newborn

Transient tachypnea of the newborn (TTN), a common abnormality in the newborn, is believed to result from delayed clearance of normal fluid from the newborn lung by the capillaries and lymphatics. It is a process more commonly observed in infants delivered by cesarean section, infants of diabetic mothers, and newborns with hypoproteinemia and hypervolemia. The onset is usually immediately after birth, and resolution should occur within 72 hours. The radiographic features include cardiomegaly, prominent vascular markings, hyperexpansion of the lungs, and ill-defined hazy to streaky infiltrates, predominantly in the bases and pleural fluid, usually in the horizontal fissure. The radiographic differentiation between TTN and CHF may be particularly difficult, as can its distinction from pneumonia.

Bronchopulmonary Dysplasia

Bronchopulmonary dysplasia (BPD) is believed to be a complication of oxygen therapy and mechanical ventilation and is most frequently a complication of the infant with HMD. It is said to occur in nearly 70% of infants treated for HMD. The onset usually blends imperceptibly with the underlying primary disease and pathologically begins within 48 to 72 hours after delivery, with resolution requiring months to years. BPD is classified into four radiographic stages that relate to prognosis, with a 40% mortality observed in stage 4. In stage 1 BPD there are fine granular infiltrates, predominantly perihilar, with air bronchograms, usually indistinguishable from those of HMD. In stage 2, there is a coarser infiltrate with focal areas of atelectasis. Stage 3 features small cystic changes together with interstitial infiltrates. Coarse cystic disease with hyperaeration characterizes stage 4 BPD. Late complications of BPD include pulmonary fibrosis, pulmonary arterial hypertension, and right ventricular hypertrophy.

Wilson-Mikity Syndrome (Pulmonary Dysmaturity)

The Wilson-Mikity syndrome is felt to overlap clinically, pathologically, and radiologically the changes of BPD. It differs from BPD in exhibiting both a later onset and absence of a history of HMD, prolonged oxygen therapy, and mechanical ventilation. The precise etiology is unclear, although pulmonary dysmaturity is felt to be a common denominator. The onset of Wilson-Mikity syndrome occurs generally when the infant is between 2 and 3 weeks of age. The prognosis is generally better than that of BPD. Roentgenographic findings are similar to those in BPD. The syndrome is rarely reported from neonatal centers at the present time.

Neonatal Pneumonias

The causes of neonatal pneumonias include infectious pneumonia, meconium aspiration, and aspiration of amniotic fluid or gastric contents.

Infectious pneumonias in the neonate are usually caused by group B streptococci. *Staphyloccus aureas, Escherichia coli, Candida* spp, herpes virus, *Listeria,* and cytomegalovirus are also occasionally observed. Predisposing conditions include prolonged maternal labor, premature rupture of the membranes, vaginal infection, amnionitis, maternal sepsis, and maternal fecal contamination at the time of delivery. The infants often will not be febrile yet exhibit respiratory distress. Septicemia is common, and mortality is high if appropriate antibiotic therapy is not initiated immediately. The clinical onset of the neonatal pneumonia is usually within the first 6 hours following delivery, and recovery is usually rapid—within 48 to 72 hours. The radiologic manifestations are usually asymmetric, patchy to diffuse fine infiltrates with air bronchograms, often with associated pleural effusions. Hyperinflation of the lungs should help to distinguish these infants from those with HMD, as does the asymmetry of the coarse, patchy infiltrates. Lobar consolidation, abscesses, and empyema are rarely seen as complicating features. However, pulmonary hemorrhage is occasionally seen.

Neonatal meconium aspiration often complicates prolonged labor or fetal distress. It is estimated that nearly 10% of amniotic fluid is meconium stained at the time of delivery, yet only 10% of these infants demonstrate respiratory distress believed to be secondary to meconium aspiration. Meconium staining is a result of fetal distress and hypoxia, which presumably induces vagal stimulation, causing in utero defecation. The aspirated meconium obstructs the bronchial tree, causing atelectasis, and initiates a reactive pneumonitis. Later, air trapping causes the appearance of marked hyperinflation. The radiographic features may be indistinguishable from those of other neonatal pneumonias. However, asymmetric air-space disease and marked hyperinflation are characteristic.

Amniotic fluid and gastric aspiration are common in the neonate. The radiographic appearance is similar to that of meconium aspiration, but marked hyperinflation is not usually seen. Since a reactive pneumonitis is not elicited, the clinical course is more benign, with resolution apparent within 72 hours after birth.

Persistent Fetal Circulation

Persistent fetal circulation (PFC) occurs as a primary or secondary process in the newborn infant. In the primary form, the neonate presents immediately following birth with hyperinflated but clear lungs and normal to diminished pulmonary vascularity, usually with cardiomegaly. Resolution commonly occurs within 48 to 72 hours. The secondary form of this abnormality is quite different radiologically and clinically. Underlying neonatal pneumonia, HMD, and aspiration or congenital abnormalities lead to increased pulmonary arterial resistance and the reopening of a patent ductus or foramen ovale, creating a right-to-left shunt. The secondary form is then more difficult to recognize roentgenographically when superimposed on the existing pulmonary disease.

Infant of a Diabetic Mother

The infant of a diabetic mother has the striking clinical appearance of macrosomia, visceromegaly, and excessive birth weight. These infants are at risk for developing HMD and congestive heart failure because of an underlying cardiomyopathy. The chest radiograph is striking in view of the child's size, with increased extrathoracic soft tissue width (the combined right and left lateral thoracic wall fat thickness should not exceed 8 mm in the normal neonate), cardiomegaly, hepatosplenomegaly, changes of congestive heart failure, and HMD. Sacral deformities in the caudal regression syndrome, renal vein thrombosis, urogenital defects, and intracranial hemorrhage may also occur.

Pulmonary Developmental Abnormalities

Pulmonary Underdevelopment

This rather broad category consists of agenesis or hypoplasia of pulmonary veins and arteries as well as bronchi and alveoli. The abnormality is usually unilateral. When bilateral, it is almost always fatal. Associated abnormalities include congenital heart disease (atrial septal defect, coarctation, PDA, tetralogy of Fallot, partial anomalous pulmonary venous return); hemivertebrae; and renal, genitourinary, and gastrointestinal anomalies. Isolated agenesis of a lobe of the lung usually involves the right upper and right middle lobes. Venolobar syndrome is virtually always right-sided, with an associated "scimitar sign" noted in one third of the cases. The scimitar sign is related to the anomalous right pulmonary vein draining to the inferior vena cava below the diaphragm, producing a curvilinear tubular density near the dextrapositioned border of the right side of the heart. The radiographic features vary with the degree of involvement but are virtually always associated with volume loss in the right lung; a small, bony hemithorax on the right side with mediastinal shift to the involved side; and overinflation of the contralateral lung in the absence of air trapping.

Cystic Adenomatoid Malformation

This is a hamartomatous pulmonary abnormality, usually unilateral, that is responsible for fetal distress based on the size of the mass lesion. In the newborn period, the mass is usually solid, as in utero fluid has not been evacuated. If the entity presents later in the child's life, it is more frequently air-filled and cystic in nature and may mimic a lung abscess, a collection of lung cysts, or even a congenital diaphragmatic hernia with bowel contents in the chest. A contralateral shift results from the mass effect.

Congenital Lobar Emphysema

This entity results from maldevelopment of the bronchi feeding a lobe or segment, with resulting hyperexpansion. As with cystic adenomatoid malformation, the initial manifestation may be a fluid-filled mass lesion that later evacuates and becomes uniformly air-filled, appearing hyperlucent. The left upper lobe is most frequently involved, followed by the right upper and middle lobes. The distinction of this condition from a pulmonary vascular sling with bronchial obstruction should be made with an esophagram, echocardiogram, and bronchoscopic study.

Diaphragmatic Hernia

Congenital herniation of the diaphragm is a neonatal emergency. The herniations most often occur on the left side, through the foramen of Bochdalek. They less frequently extend through the anterior Morgagni foramen or centrally. Since these defects occur in utero, the compressed lung is prevented from normal development and is hypoplastic. The involved hemithorax often fills with intestinal gas, and the abdomen is scaphoid, with much of its contents displaced into the affected thorax. Occasionally a fluid-filled stomach in the chest simulates a pleural effusion or other mass. The liver, spleen, or kidney may also be displaced into the thorax. Mediastinal shift is a constant feature. Once diagnosed, this condition constitutes a surgical emergency.

Tracheoesophageal Atresia

Five types of tracheoesophageal atresias occur as a result of the presumed failure of the ventral and dorsal foregut derivatives to separate in utero (Fig 1–1). Associated conditions include imperforate anus and duodenal atresia. The most common type of esophageal atresia is represented by a blind-ending proximal pouch in the proximal or midesophagus with an anomalous fistulous communication between the trachea and the lower esophagus and resulting distention of the intestines through this fistulous communication. This is the type C form, which is present in 80% to 90% of occurrences. Type A, the next most common form, is esophageal atresia with no communication between the trachea and the gastrointestinal tract (Table 1–1).

Bronchopulmonary Sequestration

Bronchopulmonary sequestrations are foregut anomalies that consist of aggregates of alveolar and bronchial tissue which normally do not communicate with the respiratory tract. They share arterial blood supply from the aorta, are most commonly seen in the posterior lower lobes, and are classically divided into intralobar and extralobar types. The intralobar type lies within the normal pleura of the lung and is drained by the pulmonary venous system. In contrast, extralobar sequestration lies outside the pleura of the lungs and drains

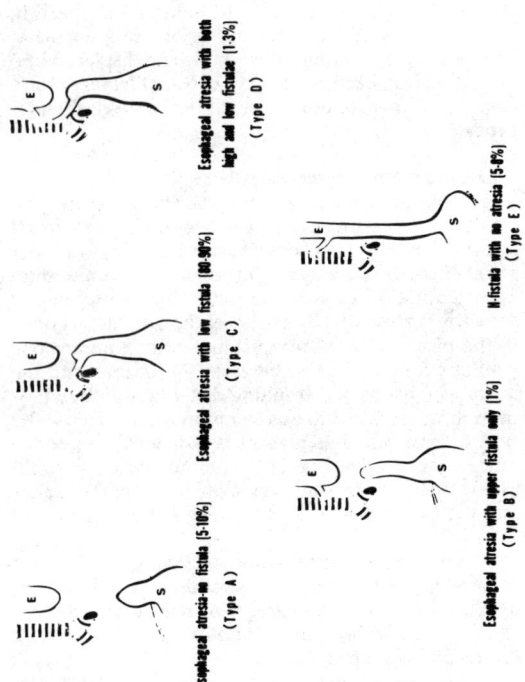

FIG 1–1.
Esophageal atresia and tracheoesophageal fistula. (From Swischuk LE: *Radiology of The Newborn and Young Infant*, ed 2. Baltimore, Williams & Wilkins, 1980. Reproduced by permission.)

TABLE 1–1.
Considerations in Evaluating the Neonatal Chest

Diagnosis*	Lung Volume*	Pleural Fluid	Heart Size	Diffuse Involvement*
HMD	↓	No	Normal	Yes
TTN	Normal to ↑	Yes	↑	Yes
BPD	Depends on stage	No	Normal	—
Wilson-Mikity	Depends on stage	No	Normal	—
Neonatal pneumonia	Variable	Yes	Normal	—
Meconium aspiration	↑	Yes	Normal or ↑	—
Massive amniotic fluid aspiration	Normal to ↑	Yes +/−	Normal to ↑	Yes
Barotrauma	↑	No	Normal	Yes
CHF	Normal to ↓	Yes +/−	↑	Yes
PFC	↑	No	↑	Yes
PDA	Variable	Yes +/−	↑	Yes
Infant of diabetic mother	Normal or ↓	No	↑	Yes
Hydrops fetalis	↓	Yes	Normal	Yes
Pulmonary underdevelopment	↓	No	Normal	Yes
Cystic adenomotoid malformation	↑	No	Normal	—

Diagnosis						
Congenital lobar emphysema	—	↑			No	Normal
Diaphragmatic hernia	—	↓			—	Normal
T-E fistula*	—	↑			—	Normal

Diagnosis	Patchy	Onset	Resolution	Comments
HMD	—	Immediate	7-10 days	Complications: BPD, PDA, barotrauma
TTN	—	Immediate	1-3 days	Ddx: CHF and pneumonia*
BPD	Yes	Immediate	Mo to yr	Four stages
Wilson-Mikity	Yes	1-4 wk	Mo to yr	Similar to BPD only delayed onset & no history of HMD or high [O₂] therapy, lower lobes
Neonatal pneumonia	Yes	0-36 hr	4-7 days	B-Strep, S. aureas, E. coli; treat immediately
Meconium aspiration	Yes	Immediate	5-10 days	Barotrauma often complicates
Massive amniotic fluid aspiration	Yes	Immediate	5-7 days	Extraventilatory air common
Barotrauma	Yes	Varies	Varies	PIE, extraventilatory air

(Continued.)

TABLE 1–1. (cont.)

Diagnosis	Patchy	Onset	Resolution	Comments
CHF	—	Varies	Varies	Numerous causes
PFC	—	Varies	2–6 days	Primary and secondary forms
PDA	—	Days 1–10	Varies	Radiograph precedes physical findings
Infant of diabetic mother	—	Immediate	3–7 days	Macrosomia, HMD, visceromegaly, obstructive murmur
Hydrops fetalis	—	Immediate	Varies	Gross edema, ascites, pleural fluid, numerous causes
Pulmonary underdevelopment	Yes	Immediate		Agenesis, aplasia, hypoplasia, venolobar bronchial stenosis, sequestration
Cystic adenomatoid malformation	Yes	Varies	Surgical	Ddx: *Staphylococcus* pneumonia, diaphragmatic hernia, congenital lobar emphysema
Congenital lobar emphysema	Yes	Varies	Surgical	Exclude pulmonary vascular sling

Diaphragmatic hernia	Yes	Varies	Surgical
T-E fistula*	Yes	Varies	Surgical	Scaphoid abdomen
				Five types

*HMD = hyaline membrane disease; TTN = transient tachypnea of the newborn; BPD = bronchopulmonary dysplasia; PFC = persistent fetal circulation; PDA = patent ductus arteriosus; Ddx = differential diagnosis; PIE = pulmonary interstitial emphysema; T-E = tracheoesophageal; ↑ = increased; ↓ = decreased.

into the caval or portal venous systems. The extralobar type is usually associated with other congenital anomalies such as absent hemidiaphragm and hypoplastic lung. Both types occasionally are associated with gastroenteric communication. The intralobar form typically is first seen later in childhood as a recurrent lower lobe pneumonia, usually on the left side. However, they may present in the neonatal period as a result of mass effect or infection.

Pulmonary Lymphangiectasia

This rare but usually fatal condition results from persistence of embryonic lymphatic drainage of the lungs. As a result of this impaired lymphatic drainage, numerous cystic and distended lymph channels develop throughout the lungs. Lymphangiectasia may be confined to the lungs or occasionally present in conjunction with congenital heart disease such as pulmonic atresia, total anomalous pulmonary venous return, or hypoplastic left heart syndrome. The initial symptoms are respiratory distress appearing shortly after birth. Radiographically the lungs appear hyperinflated, with symmetric, coarse reticulonodular opacities. Differential considerations would include aspiration, CHF and obstructed pulmonary flow with systemic collaterals.

NEONATAL CONGESTIVE HEART FAILURE

Neonatal CHF may be caused by hypoplastic left heart syndrome, interrupted aortic arch (severe coarctation), total anomalous pulmonary venous return (TAPVR) with obstruction, maternal diabetes (cardiomyopathy), volume overload such as that which occurs through a twin-to-twin intrauterine transfusion, arteriovenous malformation, placental transfusion, or a high-output state such as the child with significant anemia and intrauterine arrhythmias. Less common causes of neonatal CHF include hypoxemia, sepsis, acidosis, and hypocalcemic states. Cardiomegaly should be present in all instances except TAPVR with obstruction. Obscured pulmonary vascular structures and pleural effusions are characteristic of CHF in the newborn. The lung volumes are decreased as a result of reduced lung compliance. The onset usually is seen within the first 72 hours following birth.

MEDIASTINAL CAUSES OF NEONATAL RESPIRATORY DISTRESS

The division of the mediastinum into anterior, middle, and posterior compartments is useful for radiologic differential diagnosis. On the lateral chest radiograph, the posterior mediastinum includes masses within the area posterior to a line drawn dorsal to the thoracic vertebrae. The middle and anterior mediastinal compartments are separated by a line extending inferiorly from the manubrium parallel to the vertebral bodies. Mediastinal masses are usually detected on plain radiographs, with confirmation by fluoroscopy, ultrasound, or computed tomography (CT). Surgical exploration is essential for the definitive diagnosis and treatment of most mediastinal masses, regardless of location.

Anterior Mediastinal Masses

Variations in size of the normal thymus represent nearly all of the anterior mediastinal "masses" in the neonate but should never be responsible for respiratory distress. Sophisticated imaging studies should not be necessary to confirm the diagnosis of thymic enlargement. The thymus atrophies in response to stress and typically will then show rebound hypertrophy 4 to 8 weeks following the stressful event. Teratomas, although more commonly found in the sacrococcygeal region, are the most common of the mediastinal germ cell tumors, and are the most frequent tumor of the anterior mediastinum. They frequently are associated with respiratory distress. Calcium and fat-density material seen on CT examination support the diagnosis of teratoma; however, their absence does not exclude the diagnosis. Cystic hygromas typically arise in the posterior triangle of the neck, but approximately 10% of these benign lymphatic tumors extend into the mediastinum where they may be responsible for significant airway obstruction in the neonate. As the name implies, these lesions are typically multicystic on CT or ultrasound study.

Middle Mediastinal Masses

Traumatic and congenital middle mediastinal masses may be found in neonates. Traumatic masses are invariably secondary to iatrogenic injuries complicating the placement of central venous catheters, endotracheal tubes, or orogastric tubes and consist of blood, pus, or chyle. Most congenital masses are either gastroenteric duplications, bronchogenic cysts, or vascular anomalies. Approximately 10% to 15% of gastroenteric duplications are found in the thorax. These consist of mucosal lined cysts that result from incomplete embryologic canalization of the primitive foregut. Most commonly located adjacent to the esophagus, these lesions may also extend into the abdomen.

Bronchogenic cysts result from anomalous budding of the ventral foregut. They are lined with primitive respiratory epithelium and usually have a nonpatent communication with the tracheobronchial tree. Obstruction of the airway may be secondary to their typical subcarinal or paratracheal location.

Cardiovascular anomalies such as a double aortic arch, pulmonary artery sling, partial absence of the pericardium, and supradiaphragmatic TAPVR may be seen in neonates, producing respiratory distress. These lesions are rare and require CT scanning, echocardiography, and angiography for specific diagnosis.

Posterior Mediastinal Masses

Nearly 40% of all neonatal mediastinal masses are found in the posterior compartment and are all of neural origin, including ganglioneuromas, neuroblastomas, and neuroenteric duplications. Ganglioneuroma and neuroblastoma frequently contain calcium and are difficult to differentiate by CT scanning, although neuroblastoma may enhance inhomogeneously. The presence of adjacent rib destruction or bone metastases demonstrated by bone scan supports the diagnosis of neuroblastoma. Neuroenteric duplication cysts are so named because of the presence of primitive neural and gastrointestinal elements within the cyst. These posterior, cystic masses are associated with adjacent vertebral anomalies and are more frequently found in male infants.

CHEST WALL CAUSES OF NEONATAL RESPIRATORY DISTRESS

Thoracic wall abnormalities leading to respiratory distress or death are occasionally related to neuromuscular dysfunction and intrinsic bone dysplasias. The paralyzed thorax assumes a characteristic bell-shaped configuration, with elongation in the cephalocaudal and AP dimensions and shortening in the coronal dimension. Conditions such as amyotonia congenita, birth trauma to the cervical cord, and iatrogenic paralysis with Pavulon may be responsible for this chest wall appearance.

Many congenital syndromes are associated with chest wall anomalies. The dwarf dysplasias (e.g., thanatophoric dwarfism, asphyxiating thoracic dystrophy, and chondroectodermal dysplasia) feature short ribs with a small, mechanically ineffective chest wall. The metabolic dysplasias (e.g., hypophosphatasia and osteogenesis imperfecta) exhibit a more gracile, fragile rib which fractures easily, compromising chest wall function.

SELECTED REFERENCES

Polak JF, Kirkpatrick JA: Radiology of the newborn chest: The pulmonary air leak syndrome. *Postgrad Radiol* 1986; 6:19-44

Reid L: The lung: Its growth and remodeling in health and disease. *AJR* 1977; 129:777-788.

Singleton EB: Radiologic considerations of intensive

care in the premature infant. *Radiology* 1981; 140:291-300.

RECOMMENDED ADDITIONAL READING

Dunn V, Condon VR, Nixon GW, et al: Infants of diabetic mothers: Radiographic manifestations. *AJR* 1981; 137:123.

Goodman LR, Putman CE: Intensive care radiology, in *Imaging of the Critically Ill*. Philadelphia, WB Saunders, 1983.

Landing BJ: Congenital malformations and genetic disorders of the respiratory tract (larynx, trachea, bronchi and lungs). *Am Rev Respir Dis* 1979; 120:151.

Silverman FN: *Caffey's Pediatric X-ray Diagnosis*, ed 8. Chicago, Year Book Medical Publishers, 1985, vol II, pp 1130-1284.

Swischuck LE: *Radiology of the Newborn and Young Infant*, ed 2. Baltimore, Williams & Wilkins, 1980.

2

Pulmonary Infections

Howard Mann, M.D.

KEY CONCEPTS

1. In pneumonia, the causative organisms depend on the clinical context in which the infection occurs: (1) community-acquired pneumonia; (2) nosocomial pneumonia; (3) aspiration pneumonia; and/or (4) pneumonia in the immunocompromised host.

2. Bacterial pneumonia typically presents as a localized area of consolidation. Parenchymal necrosis, abscess formation, and empyema are important complications.

3. Viral pneumonias present as diffuse, bilateral consolidation.

4. Primary mycobacterial and fungal infections present with localized consolidation and regional lymph node enlargement.

5. In immunosuppressed transplant recipients, the most common etiologic agents are cytomegalovirus, *Pneumocystis carinii*, herpes viruses, and gram-positive cocci.

GENERAL CONSIDERATIONS

A useful approach to pulmonary infection is a consideration of the clinical context in which pneumonia is diagnosed. This, together with the patient's radiographic appearance, will enable the radiologist to suggest a limited number of possible etiologic infectious agents. The consulting physician may then be able to obtain further appropriate microbiologic, serologic, immunologic, and biochemical information from which to establish the final diagnosis.

The following four clinical groups should be differentiated: (1) community-acquired pneumonia; (2) nosocomial pneumonia; (3) aspiration pneumonia; and/or (4) pneumonia in the immunocompromised patient.

Of course, many clinical situations will be associated with an overlap between these groups, particularly in the hospitalized patient. For example, nosocomial and/or aspiration pneumonia in an immunosuppressed patient is a frequent clinical presentation in our era of aggressive treatment of malignancy with its associated prolonged survival and organ transplantation. However, this approach will be useful when the *predominant* mode of presentation is given due emphasis.

In the following overview of infectious agents responsible for the majority of pulmonary infections encountered in clinical practice in North America, the clinical context in which a particular manifestation occurs will be emphasized. Finally, an approach to the difficult problem of pulmonary infection in the immunosuppressed patient will be offered.

BACTERIAL PNEUMONIA

Gram-Positive Cocci

Pneumonia caused by gram-positive cocci—*Streptococcus pneumoniae*, *Staphylococcus aureas*, and group A beta-hemolytic streptococci—account for most bacterial community-acquired pneumonias. Of these three organisms, the pneumococcus is most often responsible for pneumonia in a previously healthy adult. However, *S. aureas* has become a very important cause of nosocomial infection in the immunosuppressed patient.

Pneumococcal Pneumonia

Instances of pneumococcal pneumonia occur sporadically, but important predisposing conditions include alcoholism, diabetes, congestive heart failure, splenectomy, and impaired immunoglobulin production (e.g., multiple myeloma).

Radiography.—The classic presentation is homogeneous lobar consolidation, but inhomogeneous consolidation affecting more than one lobe may occur. Cavitation is rare. Pleural effusions, once considered uncommon, may be seen in approximately 50% of patients, particularly if decubitus radiographs are obtained. Complete resolution of consolidation may lag considerably behind clinical improvement, and may take several weeks.

Staphylococcal Pneumonia

This is an uncommon infection, which seldom occurs as a primary disease in adults. It may follow a preceding viral influenza infection. However, as mentioned previously, it is an important cause of nosocomial pneumonia and may be a cause of aspiration pneumonia. Pneumonia secondary to staphylococcal bacteremia may occur in drug abusers (septic embolism complicating endocarditis), following septic thrombophlebitis, and as a complication of contamination of indwelling intravascular catheters.

Radiography.—In children, the classic presentation includes variable consolidation, empyema, and pneumatocele formation. In adults, variable areas of consolidation are present. Abscess formation may occur as a late development (25%), and empyema occurs in approximately 10% of patients. The hallmark of septic embolism is the appearance of nodular, cavitary opacities; pleural involvement with resultant empyema may follow inadequately treated or overwhelming embolism. Following influenza infection, secondary staphylococcal pneumonia may present as diffuse, bilateral consolidation.

Streptococcal Pneumonia

In the adult, streptococcal pneumonia is very uncommon, occurring primarily in epidemics involving military populations. In the preantibiotic era, 5% of acute pneumonias were caused by group A beta-hemolytic streptococci, resulting in high mortality.

Radiography.— Variable areas of lobular consolidation may occur. Pleural effusions are common, and empyema may occur in 50% to 70% of cases. The latter may obscure adjacent parenchymal involvement.

Aerobic Gram-Negative Organisms

Pneumonias caused by gram-negative organisms account for 20% of community-acquired pneumonias and 40% to 60% of hospital-associated pneumonias. Three methods of disease spread are:

1. Endogenous aspiration of oropharyngeal flora. Pharyngeal carriage rates of gram-negative organisms in normal subjects vary from 2% to 11%. In chronically or severely ill patients, this is increased to 60% to 70%. Colonization is also increased in patients on chronic antimicrobial therapy.
2. Exogenous aspiration of aerosolized bacterial particles from contaminated medication nebulizers, such as inhalation therapy equipment. The production of aerosols is associated with the transmission of very large numbers of organisms, mainly gram-negative bacilli. In addition, endotracheal and tracheosomy tubes allow organisms to bypass the upper respiratory tract mucociliary defense mechanism, facilitating deposition in terminal lung units.
3. Bacteremic spread to the lung from an extrathoracic source. The most common sources are the genitourinary and gastrointestinal tracts. Other sources include infected skin lesions and burns.

Pathogenesis is summarized in Table 2–1. A description of the specific pneumonias follows.

TABLE 2–1.
Pathogenesis of Aerobic Gram-Negative Pneumonias

Source	Organism
Endogenous aspiration from the nasopharynx	*Hemophilus influenzae*
	Klebsiella pneumoniae
	Pseudomonas aeruginosa
	Enterobacter spp.
	Escherichia coli
	Proteus spp.
Aerosolization of bacteria from contaminated nebulizers	*P. aeruginosa*
	Serratia marcescens
	Acinetobacter calcoaceticus
Bacteremic spread from an extrathoracic source	*E. coli*
	P. aeruginosa
	Enterobacter spp.

Hemophilus influenzae

This organism is frequently recovered from the upper respiratory tract of healthy adults and children, particularly the unencapsulated form. This form is frequently found in the mucoid sputum of chronic bronchitics, and is associated with exacerbations of bronchitis and pneumonia.

Pneumonia results from endogenous aspiration. Major predisposing factors are chronic obstructive pulmonary disease (COPD) and alcoholism.

Radiography.— Variable areas of consolidation may occur, indistinguishable from other bacterial pneumonias. Pleural involvement is not unusual, and empyema may develop early, resembling group A streptococcal infection.

Klebsiella Pneumoniae

This organism is found in the normal flora of the oral cavity and intestinal tract, and pneumonia occurs after endogenous aspiration. Most infections are acquired outside of the hospital. Elderly people in nursing homes appear to be a high-risk group.

Radiography.— The classic description of lobar consolidation in the right upper lobe with a bulging interlobar fissure is very uncommon. Frequently, several lobes are involved, and resolution may be associated with considerable volume loss, fibrosis, and pleural thickening. Cavitation and abscess formation are not uncommon.

Pseudomonas aeruginosa *Pneumonia*

This is found as a commensal organism in the oropharynx, and is frequently isolated from nebulizers and humidifiers. Aspiration from these two sources may result in pneumonia. Predisposing factors include chronic lung disease and the use of antibiotics, steroids, and immunosuppressive agents. It is an important cause of nosocomial pneumonia.

Radiography.— Extensive consolidation with necrosis and resultant cavitation is frequent. In addition, areas of infarction presenting as rounded shadows may be seen in neutropenic patients, similar to the appearance of invasive aspergillosis in this patient group.

Proteus *Pneumonia*

This infection is acquired as a result of endogenous aspiration. A high-risk group consists of alcoholics with COPD.

Radiography.—Variable areas of consolidation may occur, and abscess formation is common.

Enterobacter *Pneumonias*

Most cases follow endogenous aspiration, either in the community or hospital.

Radiography.—Multilobar consolidation may be

seen. Pleural involvement and abscess formation are reported very infrequently.

Serratia marcescens Pneumonia
This organism is generally an opportunistic agent and may be responsible for septicemia, endocarditis, and meningitis. It is an uncommon cause of pneumonia—usually nosocomial from exogenous aspiration.

Radiography.—Variable areas of consolidation may occur. Abscess formation is unusual, unlike pseudomonas pneumonia.

Escherichia coli Pneumonia
This pneumonia frequently occurs after bacteremic spread to the lung from the genitourinary and gastrointestinal tracts. Diabetes and renal parenchymal infection are two important predisposing factors.

Radiography.—Multilobar, lower lobe consolidation is usually present. Pleural effusions occur in about 50% of patients, but cavitation is uncommon.

Acinetobacter Pneumonia
This organism is widely distributed in nature, and up to 9% of people are oropharyngeal carriers. Nosocomial pneumonia occurs in patients with endotracheal tubes or tracheostomies. Community-acquired pneumonia results from endogenous aspiration, particularly in the elderly alcoholic.

Radiography.—Multilobar consolidation with complicating abscess formation and empyema may occur.

Legionella Pneumonia
Legionella pneumophila is an obligately gram-negative bacillus with fastidious requirements for growth. *Legionella* species are ubiquitous water organisms which

may be isolated from fresh-water lakes, plumbing fixtures, and air-conditioning systems. Thus, airborne transmission from such sites may lead to outbreaks of pneumonia. Pneumonia is more common in the elderly and in those with underlying cardiopulmonary disease, chronic renal failure, and diabetes. Immunosuppression with depressed cell-mediated immunity is a very significant risk factor. With rare exceptions, pathologic findings are confined to the lungs. Pontiac fever describes a nonpneumonic form of infection with multisystemic features: patients may present with fever, chills, headache, myalgia, diarrhea, arthralgia, and neurologic symptoms. Importantly, these symptoms may also accompany the pneumonic form.

Radiography.— Lobular consolidation of varying degrees is usual. Pleural effusions are common, while cavitation is rare. However, macroabscesses are found in approximately 25% of infections due to *L. micdadei* (Pittsburgh pneumonia agent).

Anaerobic Bacillary Pneumonia and Aspiration Pneumonia

Pathogenesis

In adults, the normal oropharyngeal flora is made up of both aerobic and anaerobic organisms. Anaerobic organisms demonstrate wide differences in susceptibility to oxygen, with some species growing best in reduced oxygen tensions, while others such as *Bacteroides fragilis* and peptostreptococci are killed by 10 minutes of exposure to air. Importantly, tissue breakdown results in conditions of low redox potential, enhancing growth of these organisms. The predominant pathogenesis of pneumonia is endogenous aspiration of oropharyngeal flora. Thus, conditions which predispose to aspiration are important predisposing factors.

The Aspiration Syndromes

Although this section deals with infection, it is important to appreciate that there are three well-defined aspiration syndromes: (1) aspiration of gastric acid (Mendelson's syndrome); (2) aspiration of large particles; and (3) aspiration of bacteria.

Aspiration of gastric acid results in acute lung injury manifesting as increased-permeability pulmonary edema. Aspiration of large particles may result in atelectasis of varying degrees distal to the occluded airways. Aspiration of oropharyngeal flora classically affects the gravity-dependent portions of the lungs, but minor degrees of aspiration may affect any portion of the lung.

Depending on the volume of aspirated secretions, the inherent virulence of the responsible organism and undefined host factors, the presentation varies from "uncomplicated" pneumonia through necrotizing pneumonia to lung abscess.

It is also important to appreciate the common occurrence of mixed infections associated with aspiration pneumonia as shown in Table 2–2.

Radiography.— Variable degrees of consolidation may be seen. The dependent lung regions are classically involved. The superior segments of the lower lobes are dependent in the supine position, and are frequently overlooked—behind the central pulmonary arteries on the frontal projection and overlying the thoracic spine on lateral projection

TABLE 2–2.
Infectious Agents in Aspiration Pneumonia

Clinical Group	Anaerobes Only (%)	Aerobes Only (%)	Mixed (%)
Community-acquired	59	9	31
Hospital-acquired	17	36	47

Multiple cavities are a feature of necrotizing pneumonia. A solitary lung abscess may be the presenting feature. A rounded opacity containing air or a fluid-level is the usual appearance. Empyema may be seen, particularly in association with necrotizing pneumonia.

VIRAL PNEUMONIAS

Viruses are generally considered as etiologic agents in childhood illnesses, whereas pneumonia in older children and young adults is frequently due to *Mycoplasma pneumoniae*. In adults generally, only influenzal pneumonia is a well-established cause of viral infection in civilian populations.

This section will consider viral pneumonia in adults, pneumonia as part of systemic viral disease, and viral pneumonia in the immunocompromised host.

Viral Pneumonia in Adults

Influenza

Influenza is usually a self-limited disease, with outbreaks occurring in the winter months. In general, three groups are recognized:

1. influenza infection followed by secondary bacterial pneumonia;
2. acute, progressive influenzal pneumonia; and
3. concomitant viral and bacterial infection.

Most patients fall into groups 1 and 3. *Strep. pneumoniae*, *S. aureus*, and *H. influenzae* are the most commonly isolated bacteria. Increasing age and underlying chronic cardiopulmonary disease are predisposing factors.

Adenoviruses

Sporadic adenovirus pneumonia in adults is rare; outbreaks have been described in military recruits. The disease is generally mild and self-limited. Bronchiolitis obliterans has been described as a complication of adenovirus infection, and may result in severe respiratory insufficiency.

Pneumonia as Part of Systemic Viral Disease

Measles. — Respiratory tract involvement is an integral part of the measles infection, and pulmonary consolidation may occur during uncomplicated disease. Severe, life-threatening pneumonia may occur.

Herpes Varicella-Zoster Virus. — Chickenpox remains an almost universal disease of early childhood. Varicella pneumonia is more severe as an adult infection, although a benign, self-limited infection is much more common. This pneumonia may present as small nodular opacities scattered diffusely in both lungs; these nodules may subsequently calcify.

Epstein-Barr Virus Infection. — Lung involvement has been described as part of the infectious mononucleosis syndrome, but it is not clear that the pulmonary opacities were specifically related to lung infection by this virus.

Viral Pneumonias in Immunocompromised Hosts

Cytomegalovirus

Cytomegalovirus is the single most important virus associated with pulmonary infection in the immunocompromised patient population. This is particularly common in renal, bone marrow, and cardiac transplant recipients, and in patients with acquired immune deficiency syndrome (AIDS).

Herpes Varicella-Zoster Virus

Primary infection may be devastating in immunosuppressed hosts. In addition, dissemination of the virus is not uncommon in patients with herpes zoster, particularly in association with lymphoma. However, this dissemination is usually limited to the skin.

Herpes Simplex Virus

Tracheobronchitis is uncommonly followed by pulmonary involvement. It probably represents contiguous spread or aspiration of oropharyngeal contents.

Measles

Giant cell pneumonia and encephalitis may be fatal complications of this infection in immunocompromised patients.

Radiography.— Viral pneumonia may present with varying degrees of lobular consolidation, indistinguishable from that of bacterial pneumonia. It may present as a diffuse pattern of ill-defined and small, irregular shadows, probably representing primary involvement of the interstitial compartment of the lung. In this case, it may be indistinguishable from infection due to *M. pneumonia* or *Pneumocystis pneumonia*. For example, cytomegalovirus and *Pneumocystis* infection may occur separately or concurrently in patients with AIDS, and the appearance on chest radiograph may be identical in all three instances. Another radiographic presentation is that of small nodules scattered diffusely throughout both lungs, as in varicella pneumonia.

THE ATYPICAL PNEUMONIAS

Conventionally, the organisms responsible for the so-called atypical pneumonias are *M. pneumoniae*, *Chlamydia psittaci*, and *Coxiella burnetii*. These infections more closely resemble viral infections, particularly with respect to their propensity to cause a systemic infection with many extrapulmonary manifestations. Of these, *Mycoplasma* infection is by far the most important from a clinical perspective.

Mycoplasma Pneumonia

The spectrum of pulmonary manifestations of *Mycoplasma* infection ranges from a self-limited upper respiratory tract illness to severe pneumonia. The extrapulmonary manifestations are legion and are summarized in Table 2–3.

It is important to note that *Mycoplasma* has only occasionally been demonstrated in the lungs of patients with fatal infection; thus, an immune pathogenesis has been postulated for its effect in the lung, as well as its extrapulmonary manifestations. One third to three fourths of patients develop high titers of polyclonal cold hemagglutinins.

Pulmonary Manifestations

Clinically apparent pneumonia occurs in 10% or less of cases of *Mycoplasma* pneumonia, with symptomatic pharyngotracheobronchitis occurring commonly. Several instances of the adult respiratory distress syndrome associated with *Mycoplasma* have been reported.

Radiography.—The radiographic patterns are nonspecific. Variable areas of consolidation may be seen, with either unilateral or bilateral involvement. A diffuse reticulonodular pattern may be seen, simulating that of viral pneumonia. Pleural effusions occur in up to 20% of patients. Lung abscess is very rare.

Psittacosis

This unusual respiratory infection is caused by *C. psitacci*, a common pathogen among avian species. Most human cases follow contact with psittacine birds such as parakeets and parrots, but other species may also carry the organism; thus, "Ornithosis" is a more appropriate term. After inhalation, the organism disseminates to the reticuloendothelial system and then spreads hematogenously to the lung and other organs. As with *Mycoplasma*, extrapulmonary manifestations may occur.

Radiography.—Nonspecific findings include variable areas of lobular consolidation, often perihilar in distribution. Effusions are rare. Lymph node enlargement is uncommon.

TABLE 2–3.
Extrapulmonary Involvement in *Mycoplasma* Infection

Hematologic	Autoimmune hemolytic anemia, thrombocytopenia, disseminated intravascular coagulation
Gastrointestinal	Gastroenteritis, hepatitis, pancreatitis
Musculoskeletal	Arthralgias, myalgias, polyarthritis
Dermatologic	Rashes, erythema nodosum and multiforme, Stevens-Johnson syndrome
Cardiac	Pericarditis, myocarditis, conduction defects
Neurologic	Meningitis, encephalitis, myelitis, cranial and peripheral neuropathy
Miscellaneous	Lymphadenopathy, splenomegaly, interstitial nephritis, and glomerulonephritis

Q Fever Pneumonia

In the United States, Q fever pneumonia is very uncommon, occurring mainly in farming and rural communities. The organism is rickettsia-like and is isolated from ticks. *Coxiella burnetti* is maintained in nature by animal-to-animal spread, and is inhaled by man from the heavily contaminated dust in sheep and cattle pens. Human infection is most frequently a benign illness, and extrapulmonary manifestations are not uncommon.

Radiography.—The radiographic manifestations may resemble those of viral and *Mycoplasma* pneumonia. Single, rounded opacities have been described as having a "ground-glass" appearance. Pleural effusions and lymph node enlargement are rare.

MYCOBACTERIAL INFECTIONS

Mycobacterial infections include both the tuberculous and nontuberculous mycobacterial organisms that may cause pulmonary infection. The latter are conventionally referred to as the "atypical" mycobacteria. Skin test surveys reveal that infection rates with nontuberculous mycobacteria are higher than infection rates with *Mycobacterium tuberculosis*, but the reported incidence of disease caused by these organisms is only 10% to 15% of all patients with mycobacterial disease.

Tuberculosis

Mycobacterium tuberculosis is an obligate aerobe with a high lipid content in the cell wall. The bacillus is acid-fast.

About 25,000 cases of active tuberculosis (TB) are reported each year. In about 95% of patients, clinical illness is the result of reactivation of previous disease. However, it is very important to appreciate that many adults in the United States may reach old age without previous exposure to the organism and the resultant development of cell-mediated immunity. Thus, primary TB may be found in the elderly, particularly those who live in institutions and nursing homes, and is completely overlooked when the patient is first evaluated.

Pathogenesis

A detailed understanding of the pathogenesis of this disease is necessary in order to appreciate the radiographic presentation of the different forms of pulmonary TB.

After they are inhaled, the organisms tend to accumulate in the gravity-dependent lung zones, where the initial parenchymal process ensues. *Mycobacteria* then invade the lymphatics and travel to the hilar and mediastinal lymph nodes. Hematogenous dissemination then occurs, with deposition of organisms in multiple organs. In the lung, organisms also spread to the apical regions of both lungs, providing a focus for potential reactivation.

After the development of cell-mediated immunity, "healing" may take place with the formation of parenchymal and nodal granulomas. However, viable organisms may still be present in these apparently sterile lesions, with reactivation occurring decades after the initial infection.

The Radiology of Primary and Reactivation Tuberculosis

Primary Tuberculosis.—The hallmark of primary TB is the combination of a parenchymal opacity and hilar/regional lymph node enlargement. However, as most patients are asymptomatic, this stage may pass unnoticed. Subsequent radiographs may show calcified and/or noncalcified granulomas. The combination of parenchymal and lymph node granulomas constitutes the so-called primary complex.

In some patients, the parenchymal focus is subpleural in location, and subsequent involvement of the pleural space may result in a pleural effusion that completely obscures the parenchymal focus. Thus, an important and often unappreciated presentation of primary TB is a unilateral effusion. In some patients who present with symptomatic primary TB, the only evidence of infection may be lymph node enlargement; no parenchymal opacity is discernible.

In a very small number of patients, adequate cell-mediated immunity does not develop, and progressive primary TB ensues. This appears as progressive consolidation on chest radiographs. Lastly, miliary tuberculosis describes a diffuse, bilateral micronodular pattern (nodules 1 to 2 mm in size) that represents hematogenous dissemination of organisms in the lung, reflecting an absent or severely impaired immune response.

Reactivation Tuberculosis.—Endogenous reactivation TB may occur years to decades after the primary infection. Typically, reactivation occurs in the apical segment of the upper lobes, but involvement of other segments and lobes does not exclude TB from the differential diagnosis. Parenchymal cavitation is a very common occurrence, in which case organisms are readily demonstrated in stained sputum samples. Spread of organisms may occur by way of the bronchial tree to involve other areas of both lungs. Variable areas of consolidation are a typical feature of so-called bronchogenic spread of TB. Importantly, dissemination of organisms with a nodular or micronodular pattern may occur as a result of an intercurrent disease associated with depressed cell-mediated immunity; an example is the patient with AIDS, in whom the infection may be associated with the development of the adult respiratory distress syndrome.

Complications and Other Manifestations of Pulmonary Tuberculosis

Empyema and Bronchopleural Fistula.— Infection of the pleural space may result in varying degrees of pleural fibrosis/thickening, classically with extensive calcification. A persistent, localized collection of fluid may persist in spite of extensive fibrosis, and viable organisms are often recovered from these largely unappreciated pleural collections.

Endobronchial Tuberculosis.—Although bronchial involvement and compression are commonly due to adjacent, enlarged lymph nodes, endobronchial masses occasionally occur. Patients may present with symptoms of airway obstruction.

Pulmonary Artery Erosion.—This very uncommon complication may result in fatal hemoptysis. The involved vessel has been referred to as a "Rasmussen's aneurysm."

Mycetoma Formation.—A fungus ball may develop in a parenchymal cavity caused by tuberculosis pneumonia. Hemorrhage may be the first manifestation of this complication.

Indications for Radiography in Pulmonary Tuberculosis

Although chest radiography was used extensively in the past for the detection of asymptomatic TB in the general population, a current appreciation of the epidemiology of TB and role of skin tests permits the following guidelines:

1. Routine programs of surveillance in the general community should be discontinued.
2. In asymptomatic persons with a positive tuberculin test, routine, annual chest radiography is unwarranted.
3. Patients being treated with conventional chemotherapy for TB should undergo radiography when symptoms worsen or recur, or when clinical examination suggests uncontrolled disease.
4. A mandated chest radiograph should not be a condition of employment. An initial chest radiograph may be obtained when a new employee has a positive tuberculin test.

Pulmonary Disease Caused by Nontuberculous Mycobacteria

The Runyon classification separates these organisms based on several factors including colony pigmentation and growth rates. However, since Runyon's report, more organisms have been found and studied and are not readily encompassed by this classification. Thus, each organism should be identified and defined by its own unique characteristics. In this section only the most important organisms causing pulmonary disease in man will be described.

The diagnosis of true infection by these organisms is difficult. Healthy individuals may have bacteria in their sputum without evidence of disease, but the presence of abnormal parenchymal opacities on chest radiography warrants further evaluation. In addition, disease progresses less rapidly than tuberculous infection. Nontuberculous infection may be superimposed on COPD, and may be seen in alcoholics and in elderly, debilitated patients.

Mycobacterium kansasii

This bacterium has been found predominantly in several diverse areas: Kansas City; Chicago; Texas; England; and Wales. It appears to be a disease of whites. Up to 50% of patients may be asymptomatic. Disseminated infection may occur, sometimes in association with leukemia. However, infection alone may cause a leukemoid reaction that disappears on treatment.

Radiography.—Cavitary disease involving the upper lobes is common, and is indistinguishable from tuberculosis. Thin-walled cavities with little surrounding parenchymal opacity is another presentation. Bronchogenic spread is not a feature of nontuberculous infection. Uncommonly, ill-defined nodular opacities are seen.

Mycobacterium avium-intracellulare

Generally, this infection occurs with pre-existent pulmonary and nonpulmonary diseases. These include COPD, silicosis, and malignancy. This infection has become a very important cause of pulmonary disease in patients with AIDS. It is not uncommon for the pulmonary disease to remain relatively stable without treatment and in the face of persistently positive sputum cultures.

Radiography.—Upper lobe cavitary disease is the usual presentation, and is thus indistinguishable from tuberculosis.

Mycobacterium fortuitum

This organism is a rare cause of pulmonary infection, and it is not always certain that it is responsible for the radiographic findings. It has been described in association with achalasia of the esophagus.

ACTINOMYCOSIS AND NOCARDIOSIS

Actinomyces and *Nocardia* were formerly grouped with fungi, but are now considered bacteria, with some characteristics shared with mycobacteria.

Actinomycosis

Actinomyces israelii is an anaerobic bacterium that is normally found in the oral cavity, tonsillar crypts, and more distally in the gastrointestinal tract. The presence of devitalized tissue facilitates the proliferation of this organism and the occurrence of true infection.

The most common infection is a localized process involving the tissues of the jaw and neck, which may be complicated by fistula and sinus tract formation. Pulmonary infection begins as a localized parenchymal process and, if unchecked at this stage, progresses to pleural involvement with frequent involvement of the tissues of the chest wall. In this situation, characteristic "sulfur granules" may be observed in the material obtained from the infected site.

Radiography.—As mentioned previously, focal parenchymal opacity is the initial finding. As symptoms may be absent or minimal at this time, the initial presentation may reveal localized rib or vertebral body involvement. This should always be sought for in the case of chronic infection unresponsive to initial treatment.

Nocardiosis

Nocardia asteroides and *N. brasiliensis* are soil saprophytes and are gram-positive organisms. *Nocardia* causes pulmonary infection, particularly in patients with reticuloendothelial malignancy (e.g., Hodgkin's disease). However, it may also occur in apparently immunocompetent hosts, particularly those with underlying chronic lung disease such as emphysema. Interestingly, this organism has not uncommonly been found in association with pulmonary alveolar proteinosis. Disseminated nocardial infection is another presentation of this infection.

Radiography.—Homogeneous or inhomogeneous consolidation may be seen. Cavitation may occur over days to weeks. Empyema is not an uncommon complication. In immunosuppressed patients, an important radiographic presentation is a parenchymal nodule/s which may cavitate; this presentation is indistinguishable from that seen with invasive aspergillosis.

PULMONARY FUNGAL INFECTIONS

These infections may involve both the healthy and immunocompromised host. The radiographic appearance will thus vary, and this will be emphasized in the following overview of the most common organisms responsible for infection in North America.

Among healthy individuals, three infections are most prevalent: histoplasmosis; coccidioidomycosis; and blastomycosis. The organisms are dimorphic: an infective mycelial form and a tissue yeast form may be found.

Aspergillus and *Cryptococcus* are occasional causes of

disease in the normal host. In immunosuppressed hosts, both these organisms may be responsible for disease, along with the Phycomycetes, chiefly *Mucor* species.

Histoplasmosis

Inhalation of dust-borne micronidia of *Histoplasma capsulatum* may lead to a large variety of subclinical, acute, chronic, and delayed pulmonary manifestations. In any individual, a combination of factors such as age, pre-existent parenchymal disease, immunocompetence, and other "unknown" host factors will determine which manifestation(s) will occur.

The tissue culture–positive manifestations are primary, disseminated, and chronic fibrocavitary histoplasmosis. The tissue culture–negative forms are calcified or noncalcified histoplasma granulomas, and granulomatous fibrosing mediastinitis. These will be described individually.

Histoplasma capsulatum grows best in soil contaminated by the droppings of birds, such as chickens, and by bat guano. It is most prevalent in the river valleys of the Mississippi and Ohio rivers, but many other areas in temperate and tropical climactic zones harbor the organism. The micronidia become airborne when the soil in which they are found is disturbed, and are inhaled into the distal lung units.

Primary Pulmonary Histoplasmosis

After inhalation, the tissue yeast form undergoes lymphohematogenous dissemination. As with TB, a granulomatous response occurs with concurrent parenchymal and nodal involvement. Caseation necrosis is followed by healing associated with fibrosis and calcification. In the large majority of cases, the primary infection is asymptomatic.

Radiography.—If radiographs are obtained during the acute symptomatic phase, focal parenchymal opacity associated with hilar and/or mediastinal lymph node enlargement may be seen. As with TB, only lymph node enlargement may be identified. In the case of inhalation of a massive number of organisms, as may occur with persons who explore underground caves, a diffuse, multinodular pattern is common. In these previously exposed persons, healing occurs without the formation of calcified granulomas, and lymph node enlargement is not a feature. Pleural effusion accompanying the primary infection is rare.

Disseminated Histoplasmosis

Infants, young children, and the immunosuppressed patient may manifest progressive, life-threatening dissemination. In this situation, the extrapulmonary manifestations are prominent with hepatosplenomegaly and generalized lymphadenopathy. Other clinical features may include chronic meningitis, adrenal insufficiency, subacute endocarditis, and mucocutaneous lesions.

Radiography.—The radiograph may be normal, or lymph node enlargement may be present, with variable parenchymal involvement.

Chronic Fibrocavitary Histoplasmosis

The pathogenesis of this form is very uncertain. Some investigators feel that this represents reinfection, rather than endogenous reactivation as occurs with TB. The initial process fails to resolve, and progressive upper lobe cavitary disease with severe fibrosis and volume loss occurs. Bronchogenic spread to the dependent parts of the lower lobes may also ensue.

Radiography.— Upper lobe parenchymal opacity with cavitation and progressive volume loss is common. Thus, this appearance may not be distinguishable from reactivation TB and its sequela.

Histoplasma Granulomas

These represent the "healed" form of this disease, and may occasionally present as a solitary, noncalcified pulmonary nodule.

Radiography.—The typical appearance is that of multiple, bilateral calcified nodules, with prominent splenic involvement. In the case of a solitary nodule suspected to be a histoplasmoma, other imaging procedures may be used to elicit the presence of benign calcification, such as low-kV(p) spot radiographs, and conventional or computed tomography.

Granulomatous Fibrosing Mediastinitis

This unusual, progressive form of the disease may result in extensive mediastinal fibrosis with compression and occlusion of many mediastinal structures such as vessels, bronchi, trachea, esophagus, and pericardium. Symptoms and signs will depend on the structures involved. Possible abnormalities include superior vena cava syndrome, volume loss of varying degrees, dysphagia, dyspnea due to tracheal involvement, hemoptysis, infarction, and pericardial constriction. An unusual presentation is occlusion of a bronchus by a calcified broncholith, the result of lymph node erosion through the wall of a bronchus.

Radiography.—Calcified lymph nodes may be seen on chest radiographs. Computed tomography is the most efficacious means of evaluating this manifestation of the disease, and enables visualization of all important mediastinal structures with one examination.

Coccidioidomycosis

This disease is endemic in the Southwestern U.S., parts of Southern Utah, and Northern Mexico (Lower Sonoran Life Zone). However, *Coccidioides immitis* is seen in many other parts of the U.S. and around the world; its high rate of infectivity and its transmission by transcontinental travellers has led to the descriptor "flying arthrospore." The organism germinates in soil as an infectious arthrospore; while in tissues it takes the form of an endosporulating spherule. The spectrum of coccidioidal infection consists of three major pulmonary syndromes: (1) primary coccidioidomycosis; (2)

disseminated (micronodular) coccidioidomycosis; and (3) progressive and persistent cavitary pulmonary coccidioidomycosis.

Primary Coccidioidomycosis

In endemic regions, 60% of infections are asymptomatic. It is generally a self-limited disease, presenting with constitutional symptoms and a nonproductive cough. In 10% to 20% of cases, there are associated hypersensitivity skin lesions such as erythema nodosum and multiforme, in addition to a polyserositis and polyarthritis.

Radiography.— Initially, variable areas of consolidation are seen, occasionally with hilar lymph node enlargement. Areas of consolidation may resolve in one area while new areas of consolidation appear elsewhere. Acute cavitation may then occur to leave thin- or thick-walled cavities, a feature very uncommon in other pneumonias, particularly in the atypical or viral pneumonias. Pleural effusions are not uncommon, probably due to contiguous spread from an adjacent subpleural focus.

Chronic Progressive Coccidioidal Pneumonia

Patients with this form of the disease generally have a well-defined history of primary infection, which does not resolve in the usual fashion. The course is unpredictable, but appears to be dependent on the presence of severe pre-existent disease, particularly those associated with an immunosuppressed state. In those patients who die from this manifestation, the majority have no evidence of extrapulmonary disease. Importantly, this manifestation closely mimics reactivation TB, with chronic recovery of the organism from the sputum. This form accounts for approximately 1% of cases.

Radiography.— Bilateral, apical fibrocavitary disease is present. The rate of progression is very variable, but significant fibrosis and volume loss may occur.

Persistent Cavitary Disease

Uncommonly, patients may develop cavitation in association with the primary infection, which does not subsequently resolve. The cavity may follow an asymptomatic infection, and may thus be discovered incidentally. The cavity is usually single and may be thin- or thick-walled. The subsequent course is unpredictable, but complete healing occurs in most cases, although this may take several years. Most nonresolving cavities tend to be asymptomatic or associated with intermittent, mild hemoptysis. Infrequent complications of this situation include colonization of the cavity by another organism (*Aspergillus* or pyogenic bacteria) and rupture of a subpleural cavity into the pleural space, with resultant pyopneumothorax.

Disseminated Coccidioidomycosis

This represents hematogenous dissemination of the organism to many body sites, and is prone to occur in diabetics and immunosuppressed patients. Rapidly progressive respiratory failure may ensue.

Radiography.— A miliary pattern resembling miliary TB may be seen.

Pulmonary Coccidioidoma

This may present as a calcified or noncalcified solitary pulmonary nodule. It may be up to 5 cm in size. When discovered incidentally, a history of travel to an endemic area should be sought. This lesion is not simply a sterile residue of a past infection, as *C. immitis* is often identifiable in the gelatinous or necrotic center. As with other solitary pulmonary nodules, percutaneous biopsy may be performed in an attempt to establish the diagnosis.

North American Blastomycosis

Blastomycosis is caused by the dimorphic fungus *Blastomyces dermatitidis*. This organism is endemic in the southeastern and midwestern U.S., where the reservoir is presumed to be in the soil. Infection occurs through inhalation, and most primary infections are asymptomatic and self-limited.

Hematogenous dissemination of the organism may occur, and subsequent skin and bone involvement may be prominent, distinguishing this infection from the other deep mycoses.

Radiography.— The usual finding is focal consolidation, which may be nodular in configuration. Cavitation is uncommon. Adjacent rib destruction may be present, representing hematogenous dissemination to bone.

Aspergillosis

The infecting organism, usually *Aspergillus fumigatus*, is a dimorphic soil fungus worldwide in distribution. The organism is a common finding in the sputum of normal individuals, with infection resulting from an altered host immune response or other predisposing factors.

In general, four distinct manifestations of infection may be considered: (1) fungus ball (mycetoma) formation; (2) invasive aspergillosis; (3) semi-invasive aspergillosis; or (4) allergic bronchopulmonary aspergillosis.

Mycetoma

Formation of a fungus ball occurs within a pre-existent cavity, most commonly the result of tuberculosis, sarcoidosis, and bullous emphysema. This situation is usually undetected unless the patient presents with hemoptysis, which may be severe and necessitate curative surgical resection.

Radiography.— An opacity is present within a thin-walled cavity; this opacity is often seen in the dependent portion of the cavity, and shifts with changes in patient positioning. A thin crescent of air will be seen around the fungus ball when it almost fills the entire cavity.

Invasive Aspergillosis

This manifestation occurs in the immunosuppressed host. In particular, patients with hematologic malignancy and granulocytopenia are at high risk. Prolonged antibiotic and high-dose steroid therapy are other predisposing factors. Pulmonary involvement may be but one focus in a pattern of disseminated visceral disease.

Radiography.— The classic radiographic manifestation is the appearance of nodular opacities, with the formation of an air-crescent sign as a result of vascular invasion and focal lung infarction/necrosis. Thus, this differs from mycetoma formation described earlier, and invasive aspergillosis should be suspected in the appropriate clinical situation even before air-crescent formation within a nodule occurs. Finally, diffuse, rapidly progressive consolidation may be seen in invasive, disseminated aspergillosis.

Semi-invasive Aspergillosis

This term has been coined to describe formation of a mycetoma within an area of cavitation subsequent to focal parenchymal infection and necrosis caused by the *Aspergillus* organism itself. Persons at risk are alcoholics, those with malignancy, the elderly debilitated patient, and those with a radiation-damaged lung. Cavitation and subsequent mycetoma formation is a chronic process, unlike the situation characteristic of invasive aspergillosis.

Radiography.— Focal consolidation is seen initially, followed by a variable time interval before cavitation and fungus-ball formation occurs. Generally, an irregular cavity appears within an area of consolidation, followed by further excavation into a thin-walled cavity containing a growing fungus ball.

Allergic Bronchopulmonary Aspergillosis

This manifestation occurs primarily in chronic asthmatics in association with bronchial mucus-plugging, bronchial dilatation, peripheral eosinophilia, elevated levels of IgE, and skin hypersensitivity to the *Aspergillus* antigen. The organism is usually readily seen in expectorated mucus plugs. If patients are not appropriately treated with steroids, progressive parenchymal fibrosis may follow repeated infective episodes.

Radiography.— The key to the radiographic diagnosis is the presence of tubular shadows caused by dilated, mucus-filled bronchi. Occasionally, a "cluster of grapes" appearance may be seen in cases of severe, cystic bronchial dilatation. Variable areas of consolidation may be seen, which resolve to be followed by the appearance of consolidation in other regions of the lung. Areas of atelectatic lung may occur proximal to bronchial obstruction by mucus plugs.

Cryptococcosis

The unimorphic fungus *Cryptococcus neoformans* is found in the soil worldwide. A major environmental reservoir is birds, particularly pigeons in an urban setting. Inhalation is often followed by dissemination, with cerebral and meningeal involvement a prominent complication. Infection may occur in the normal host, but most cases of dissemination occur in persons with depressed cell-mediated immunity.

Radiography.— The radiograph may be normal, even in the presence of disseminated visceral disease and cerebral/meningeal involvement. Nodular peripheral opacities may occur, with occasional cavitation. A relatively uncommon presentation is focal consolidation.

Phycomycosis

This is caused by a variety of Phycomycetes, including species of *absidia*, *rhizopus*, and *mucor*, the last of which is by far the most common agent involved. These are soil fungi, which are inhaled in the form of spores. This disease is characteristically an opportunistic infection, occurring particularly in persons with hematologic malignancy, in the setting of chronic steroid therapy and in diabetics. In the latter group, involvement of the paranasal sinuses and orbits is a relatively common finding.

Radiography.—Focal consolidation may be seen, and a very suggestive presentation takes the form of solitary or multiple nodules which may cavitate. As with invasive aspergillosis, this represents focal infarction and necrosis.

CANDIDIASIS

Candida is a common saprophyte of the upper respiratory tract, and may be responsible for opportunistic infection in the appropriate clinical setting. In this circumstance, there is often evidence for involvement of other sites such as the oropharynx and esophagus, and the genitourinary tract.

Radiography

Focal consolidation and ill-defined nodular opacities may be seen. In severe cases, diffuse consolidation may be present, indistinguishable from other causes of extensive infection.

PROTOZOA

Infections caused by two organisms are relatively common, particularly in situations associated with depressed cell-mediated immunity: *P. carinii* and *Toxoplasma gondii*.

Pneumocystis carinii

This diffuse pulmonary parenchymal infection occurs predominantly in the following patient groups and situations: patients with AIDS; transplant patients; and those on chronic steroid therapy. Patients often present with fever, nonproductive cough, and hypoxemia.

Radiography.—Findings vary from a subtle increase in nonvascular shadows to diffuse consolidation. Pathologically, there is often a prominent interstitial pneumonia, with progression to alveolar exudation and hyaline membrane formation. A very rare manifestation is the occurrence of ill-defined nodular shadows.

Toxoplasma gondii

Pulmonary involvement is generally only a feature in disseminated disease, occurring in the immunosuppressed patient. There is commonly evidence for central nervous system and skin involvement.

Radiography.—The appearance is similar to infection with *Pneumocystis*, with diffuse consolidation.

THE IMMUNOSUPPRESSED HOST: A GUIDE TO PREDOMINANT PATHOGENS IN SPECIFIC CLINICAL SITUATIONS

As mentioned previously, the radiographic presentation must be integrated with an appreciation of the organisms most likely to be responsible for pulmonary infection in any given clinical situation. Such information is summarized in Table 2–4.

CHEST RADIOGRAPHY AND PATTERN RECOGNITION IN THE IMMUNOCOMPROMISED HOST

The appreciation of a predominant pattern on the chest radiograph in the immunocompromised host may be helpful in limiting the range of diagnostic possibilities, particularly when combined with the situational information summarized in Table 2–4.

The following list of broad categories should always be used with circumspection; mixed infections may occur, and diffuse parenchymal disease may be the result of associated noninfectious causes such as drug toxicity, hemorrhage, extension of tumor, and so-called non-

TABLE 2–4.
Predominant Pathogens in Specific Diseases and Therapeutic States*

Disease/Therapy	Specific Deficiency	Predominant Infections (pathogen)
Chronic lymphocytic leukemia; multiple myeloma	Impaired gamma globulin synthesis	*Pneumococci, Hemophilus influenzae,* meningococci, *Streptococcus, Staphylococcus, Pseudomonas aeruginosa,* some viruses, *Giardia*
Hodgkin's disease	Suppressor monocytic cells	*Cryptococcus, Listeria, Toxoplasma, Mycobacterium, Legionella,* herpes varicella-zoster, *Salmonella, Brucella, Strongyloides*
Acute leukemia	Neutropenia	Gram-negative bacilli, gram-positive cocci, *Candida, Aspergillus*
Hairy cell leukemia	Monocytopenia, impaired lymphocyte function	*Mycobacterium, Toxoplasma,* DNA viruses
Transplant recipient	Increased activity of suppressor T lymphocytes	Gram-positive cocci, *Pneumocystis,* cytomegalovirus, herpes vari-

		cella-zoster, herpes simplex virus
Adrenal corticosteroids	Multiple	Adversely affects all types of infection. Especially predisposes to *Aspergillus*, *Pneumocystis*
Splenectomy	Impaired antibody production to new antigens, tuftsin deficiency	Gram-positive cocci, *Hemophilus influenzae*, meningococci
Cancer chemotherapy	Multiple	Gram-negative bacilli, gram-positive cocci, *Candida* (usually localized, less frequently disseminated)

*From Bodey GP: Infection in cancer patients. *Am J Med* 81:1986; 81(suppl 1A):11-26. Reproduced by courtesy of the author.

specific interstitial pneumonitis, the last refering to histologic findings on open-lung biopsy in up to 38% of patients in this clinical setting.

1. Focal, segmental, and lobar consolidation. In this group, gram-negative bacilli constitute the most common etiologic agents. Cavitation and abscess formation may occur.
2. Nodular opacities with/without cavitation. Fungal infections predominate when this pattern is present. *Nocardia* is a bacterial pathogen that should always be considered.
3. Diffuse parenchymal opacity. The most common agents in this group are the viruses and protozoa, particularly *P. carinii*. Of the viruses, the most common are cytomegalovirus, herpes zoster, and herpes simplex.

SELECTED REFERENCES

Bartlett JG, O'Keefe P, Tally FP, et al: Bacteriology of hospital-acquired pneumonia. *Arch Intern Med* 1986; 146:868.

Bodey GP: Infection in cancer patients. *Am J Med* 1986; 81(suppl 1A):11.

Curry WA: Human nocardiosis. *Arch Intern Med* 1980; 140:818.

Cush R, Light RW, George RB: Clinical and roentgenographic signs of blastomycosis. *Chest* 1976; 69:345.

DeBoer Unger J, Rose HD, Unger GF: Gram-negative pneumonia. *Radiology* 1973; 107:283.

De Lorenzo LJ, Huang CT, Maguire GP, et al: Roentgenographic patterns of *Pneumocystis carinii* pneumonia in 104 patients with AIDS. *Chest* 1987; 91:323.

Drutz D, Catanzaro A: Coccidioidomycosis: State of the art. *Am Rev Respir Dis* 1978; 117:559 (Part I); 117:727 (Part II).

Edelstein PH, Meyer RD: Legionnaire's disease. *Chest* 1984; 85:114.

Feigin DS: Nocardiosis of the lung: Chest radiographic findings in 21 cases. *Radiology* 1986; 159:9.

Flynn MW, Felson B: The roentgen manifestations of thoracic actinomycosis. *AJR* 1970; 110:707.

Gefter WB, Weingrad TR, Epstein DM, et al: Semi-invasive pulmonary aspergillosis: A new look at the spectrum of aspergillus infections in the lung. *Radiology* 1981; 140:313.

Goodwin RA, Des Prez RM: Histoplasmosis: State of the art. *Am Rev Respir Dis* 1978; 117:929.

Johanson WG Jr, Harris GD: Aspiration pneumonia, anaerobic infections, and lung abscess. *Med Clin North Amer* 1980; 64:385.

Kantor HG: The many radiologic facies of pneumococcal pneumonia. *AJR* 1981; 137:1213.

Miller WT: Pulmonary infections, in Taveras JM, Ferrucci JT (eds): *Radiology, Diagnosis-Imaging-Intervention*. Philadelphia, JB Lippincott Co, 1986, vol. 1.

Niederman MS (ed): *Clinics in Chest Medicine (Respiratory Infections)*. Philadelphia, WB Saunders Co, 1987.

Ognibene FP, Pass HI, Roth JA, et al: Role of imaging and interventional techniques in the diagnosis of respiratory disease in the immunocompromised host. *J Thorac Imag* 1988; 3(2):1.

Palmer PED: Pulmonary tuberculosis—usual and unusual radiographic manifestations. *Semin Roentgenol* 1979; 14:204.

Peters SG, Prakash UBS: *Pneumocystis carinii* pneumonia. *Am J Med* 1987; 82:73.

Pierce AK, Sanford JP: Aerobic gram-negative bacillary pneumonias. *Am Rev Respir Dis* 1974; 110:647.

Putman CE, Curtis AM, Simeone JF, et al: Mycoplasma pneumonia: Clinical and radiographic patterns. *AJR* 1975; 124:417.

Wolinsky E: Nontuberculous mycobacteria and associated diseases. *Am Rev Respir Dis* 1979; 119:107.

3
Neoplastic Diseases of the Thorax
David G. Bragg, M.D.

KEY CONCEPTS

1. Destructive rib lesions are usually malignant and most frequently are of metastatic origin.
2. The most common benign rib lesions are enchondroma and fibrous dysplasia.
3. Mediastinal lesions are virtually all surgical problems.
4. Thymomas are virtually nonexistent in patients under 20 years of age.
5. Posterior mediastinal tumors are "always" of neurogenic origin.
6. There are no "pathognomonic radiographic features" of lung cancer.

CHEST WALL NEOPLASMS

Primary neoplasms of the chest wall are uncommon. Their radiographic characteristics are similar, with a destructive rib lesion and large surrounding soft tissue mass. Non-Hodgkin lymphomas involving the thoracic cage will usually mimic those changes of a Ewing sarcoma. Metastatic rib lesions are the most common cause of destructive rib lesions, regardless of patient age.

The two most common benign rib lesions are enchondromas and fibrous dysplasia (Table 3–1). Enchondromas often will contain a matrix of punctate

TABLE 3–1.
Neoplasms of Ribs

Benign
    Enchondroma (matrix calcified)
    Fibrous dysplasia (expanded, ground-glass texture)
    Osteocartilaginous exostosis
    Paget's disease
    Brown tumor (hyperparathyroidism)

Malignant
    Primary tumors
        Ewing's sarcoma
        Chondrosarcomas
        Non-Hodgkin's lymphomas
        Askin tumors (neuroepithelial neoplasm)
        Malignant fibrous histiocytoma (low-grade sarcoma, chest wall)
        Myeloma, plasmacytoma

    Metastatic tumors and multiple myeloma—differential considerations
        Callus, healing rib fracture
        Congenital deformity (bifid/fused)
        Radiation bone injury
        Metabolic bone disease

calcifications whereas fibrous dysplasia more often has a uniform texture, stated to be like "ground glass" in appearance. Osteocartilaginous exostoses may project centrally and mimic a lung mass. These lesions virtually all arise from the anterior rib margins, near the costochondral junctions. The complications of rib fractures may occasionally mimic a more destructive neoplastic lesion.

Radiography

If an extrapleural soft tissue mass is evident surrounding the destructive process on ordinary radiographs, the lesion will either be a primary bone tumor, multiple myeloma, or a lymphoma, usually a non-Hodgkin lymphoma. The uncommon benign rib lesions will be found to be contained by an intact cortex and will not have a surrounding soft tissue mass. Low kilovolt (peak) [kV(p)] plain films in the anteroposterior and oblique projections are necessary to search for suspected rib neoplasms as conventional high kV(p) chest films obscure bone detail.

PLEURAL NEOPLASMS

Benign pleural neoplastic lesions are extremely uncommon. The most common benign neoplasms are localized fibrous mesothelioma and pleural lipoma. The more frequent examples of apparent pleural "mass lesions" are merely accumulations of fat in obese patients or those on corticosteroid therapy. Occasionally, blood can organize in the pleural compartment following a long-standing pneumothorax, leaving a fibrin ball which may appear pedunculated and move with change in patient position. Loculated fluid in the pleural compartment may mimic a mass lesion; however, there are usually other manifestations of pleural fluid to suggest this diagnosis. Fat does not appear as lucent when in contrast with aerated lung, yet it always appears in a typical location along the lower lateral aspect of the intercostal spaces on the posteroanterior radiograph, which may mimic pleural thickening.

Malignant pleural tumors are usually of metastatic origin. More frequently, pleural fluid represents the only manifestation of the presence of an intrapleural metastatic process, as chest films will usually not reveal the metastatic tumor itself. The metastatic deposits tend to be microscopic yet stimulate the production of pleural fluid, which is usually positive for malignant cells when analyzed. Exceptions to this statement include effusions associated with intrathoracic lymphomas, which are usually secondary to the presence of tumor in sites other than the pleural compartment.

Mesothelioma is the most common primary tumor of the pleural compartment and is virtually always associated with significant exposure to asbestos. The diagnosis of mesothelioma is difficult, both clinically and radiologically. The radiographic manifestations of asbestos-related pleural disease overlap those of mesothelioma and include pleural plaques, pleural effusions, and enlarging pleural-based mass lesions. Calcifications within pleural plaques, particularly when bilateral, document the diagnosis of asbestos-related pleural disease. Malignant pleural mesotheliomas rarely calcify. These neoplasms usually extend along the pleural surfaces to encase the involved lung. They uncommonly extend to the chest wall structures. Associated pleural effusions are frequent but are most often cytologically negative for diagnostic cells. Computed tomographic (CT) scanning forms the basis for suggesting the diagnosis and preoperatively staging the patient.

Radiography

A pleural effusion will be the most common presenting manifestation suggesting an underlying malignant pleural tumor, either of primary or metastatic origin. Pleural involvement of metastatic origin is usually limited to the presence of an effusion on plain films. The tumor deposits are usually microscopic and not visible even on more sophisticated imaging techniques such as CT scanning. Tumors that involve the peritoneal surface or liver may occasionally extend directly to involve the pleural compartment, through the diaphragm. In these instances, a right-sided effusion, occasionally with a pleural-based mass lesion may be seen contiguous with the dome of the right hemidiaphragm. Primary pleural tumors are uncommon. Most such neoplasms will be malignant mesotheliomas that will be associated with a history of asbestos exposure.

The differentiation between asbestos-pleural plaques and malignant mesotheliomas may be difficult and often will be based on interval growth of the "pleural plaque," with extension to cover the ipsilateral pleural surface. CT scans are the primary means of exploring the pleural compartment in the patient suspected of having a pleural neoplasm.

MEDIASTINUM

Mediastinal neoplasms must be discussed by compartment, as summarized in Table 3–2. The initial diagnosis is usually a result of detection with plain chest radiography. The basis of determining the mediastinal location for a tumor has been defined by Heitzman as fulfilling three criteria: a very sharp interface of the tumor and the adjacent lung caused by the investment of the lesion by both layers of pleura; an obtuse angle of the margin of the neoplasms with the analogy of a "marble under a rug"; and displacement of or involvement with known mediastinal structures such as the esophagus, trachea, or contiguous blood vessels.

The superior mediastinal compartment is almost the sole province of enlargement of or neoplasms involving the thyroid or parathyroid glands. Rarely will parathyroid adenomas assume sufficient size to displace normal mediastinal structures or distort a mediastinal contour on a chest study. Substernal enlargement of the thyroid gland frequently does occur and may escape detection during a cursory physical examination. Such lesions displace but do not narrow the trachea unless invasion has occurred through the wall of the trachea. The more common benign enlargements of the thyroid gland detected on a chest radiograph will occupy the superior mediastinum, yet their center of origin should not extend below the level of the aortic arch for embryologic reasons. The anlage of the thyroid gland reaches the mediastinum by accompanying arch 4; therefore, the vector of origin of a superior mediastinal

TABLE 3-2.
Mediastinal Neoplasms: Compartmental Location and Incidence*

Mediastinal Compartment	Type of Tumor	Incidence (%)
Superior mediastinum	Endocrine tumors (thyroid, parathyroid, carcinoid)	5
Anterior mediastinum	Thymoma	19
	Lymphoma	17
	Germ cell tumors	13
	Mesenchymal tumors	9
	Primary carcinomas	4
Posterior mediastinum	Neurogenic tumors	31
		100

*From Armstrong JD II, Bragg DG: Thoracic neoplasms, in *Oncologic Imaging.* New York, Pergamon Press, 1985, p 167. Reproduced by permission.

mass of thyroid origin should be at or above the level of the aortic arch. Calcifications uncommonly can be seen within a thyroid mass and be associated either with a benign or malignant thyroid lesion. CT examination of thyroid neoplasms with contrast-material enhancement will show a connection with the parent thyroid gland in the neck, prolonged and often delayed contrast enhancement, and location of the gland between the esophagus and trachea. CT scanning is also critical in the location and verification of ectopic mediastinal parathyroid adenomas in the patient with clinical findings consistent with hyperparathyroidism. It has recently been shown that T2-weighted magnetic resonance (MR) images may be the most effective way yet to detect the presence of ectopic parathyroid adenomas.

The inferior margin of the superior mediastinum extends from the angle of Louis to T-4. Arbitrarily, we will define the anterior mediastinum as extending from the floor of the superior mediastinum to the diaphragm with the anterior border of the heart forming the dorsal margin. Virtually all tumors in the anterior mediastinum are surgical lesions and include the four "T's" (thymoma, teratoma, thyroid neoplasms, and tumors of lymphoid origin). Thymomas rarely occur in patients under the age of 20, so enlargements of the thymic gland can be considered benign except in those uncommon examples where a lymphoma infiltrates the thymic gland or a germ cell tumor is found to involve this structure. In infants and young children, the thymic gland may be found to be enlarged and rapidly undergo involution during times of stress.

The radiologic evaluation of the anterior mediastinum should begin with the conventional chest radiograph where the lateral view will usually show a water-density mass filling the anterior mediastinum, obliterating the normal triangle of fat which normally characterizes this region. In young adult women, this normally lucent area may be opacified by the axillary tail of the breast superimposed on this region on the lateral film with the patient's arms extended over her head. In the older individual, atherosclerotic aortic changes may superimpose the ascending and arch regions of the aorta into the structures of the anterior mediastinum. If an anterior mediastinal tumor is suspected, CT or MR imaging should be conducted to evaluate this region. Certain imaging characteristics may lead one to suspect a teratomatous tumor, particularly calcifications within ectodermal components of this lesion, resembling teeth or dystrophic calcifications. Up to 25% of teratomatous lesions may be behaviorally malignant, so these lesions should be surgically managed.

To understand the lymphomas requires an appreciation of their origins, common cytopathologic features, and classification. Hodgkin's disease exhibits a more predictable clinical and radiologic course, and the pathologic study and classification have been more stable over the years. The four pathologic types of Hodgkin's lymphomas are summarized in Table 3–3. Since Hodgkin's disease has a bimodal age of presentation, the more common patient will be the late-teenage or early 20-year-old individual with a nodular sclerosing histologic pattern. This histologic type is virtually always associated with mediastinal disease, usually in the anterior mediastinal compartment. Intrathoracic disease is less frequently seen with the other three histologic types of Hodgkin's disease. The disease progresses through echelons of the mediastinum so that lung parenchymal disease should not occur in the absence of hilar or mediastinal involvement. To reinforce this rule, an individual with no hilar or mediastinal Hodgkin's disease presenting with a parenchymal abnormality, one should assume that the lung parenchymal lesion is other than Hodgkin's. The bulky mediastinal masses which often characterize the patient with a nodular sclerosing Hodgkin's lymphoma may slowly regress following appropriate therapy, leaving an abnormal mediastinal compartment for some time. Hodgkin's disease rarely involves the lung parenchyma

TABLE 3-3.
Rye Classification of Hodgkin's Disease*

Histologic Type	Estimated Frequency (%)	
	Adult	Child
Lymphocyte predominance	10	10
Nodular sclerosis	75	65
Mixed cellularity	15-20	20
Lymphocytic depletion	10	1

*Modified from Castellino RA: *Radiology* 1986; 159:305.

as a primary, extranodal site of disease in contrast to non-Hodgkin lymphoma.

In contrast to Hodgkin's disease, the non-Hodgkin lymphomas (NHLs) represent a very heterogeneous spectrum of neoplasms with great variability in their clinical presentation, radiologic patterns of disease, course, and prognosis as well as treatment strategy. It is now felt that virtually all NHLs are neoplasms of lymphocytes and their derivatives, with the different pathologic expressions representing different stages in lymphocyte development and/or transformation. The spectrum of lymphoid neoplasms classified as NHLs are dynamic, with low-grade NHLs often evolving to higher grades during the course of the disease. The newer immunologic classifications for the lymphomas subdivide them into two arms: T- and B-lymphocytes. They also define lymphomas as clonal proliferations and assume that the more aggressive, malignant neoplasms are derived from a single clone, whereas the benign lymphoid proliferations are polyclonal in origin. Immunoperoxidase staining allows the immunologic classification of the neoplasms as being either monoclonal or polyclonal, and specific cell surface antigen characterization allows one to determine whether they are of T- or B-cell origin.

The pathologic spectrum of pulmonary lymphocytic infiltrates is a subject of considerable debate and controversy. The pathologist is challenged to separate these lesions into the variety of small lymphocytic infiltrates or nonmalignant lymphoid disorders from true non-Hodgkin lymphomas. It is now felt that the extranodal, nonmalignant lymphoid disorders share many similar radiologic qualities, represented by either infiltrates or mass lesions in the absence of hilar or mediastinal lymphadenopathy. These include lymphocytic interstitial pneumonitis, pseudolymphoma, and lymphoid granulomatosis. Many of the examples of pseudolymphoma and some lymphocytic interstitial pneumonias are monoclonal by immunologic staining, and hence are true NHLs. There are also some primary lymphoid disorders that are nonmalignant, including reactive lymph node enlargements caused by either specific infectious organisms or such systemic diseases as systemic lupus erythematosus, infectious mononucleosis, Castleman's disease (giant lymph node hyperplasia), and angioimmunoblastic lymphadenopathy.

The true NHL lesions have been the subject of numerous pathologic classifications schemes. The most recent is the Working Formulation, a compromise morphologic classification dividing the individual tumors into three grades: low, intermediate, and high. The low-grade histologic pattern more frequently is disseminated at diagnosis even though the patient often is asymptomatic and the disease course is indolent. They frequently evolve or differentiate into a high-grade lesion. In contrast, the high-grade lymphomas are more frequently localized, often the type of NHL is found in an extranodal site, and these tumors are more amenable to treatment. Our staging effort should primarily address the high-grade lesions, as they are the ones the oncologist will be more interested in aggressively treating.

A similar staging system is used for both Hodgkin's disease and the NHLs. This four-stage system is summarized in Table 3–4.

The different types of lymphomas share more similarities than differences as represented by the various imaging studies. Hodgkin's lymphomas are almost exclusively mediastinal nodal tumors on presentation, with the anterior mediastinal compartment most frequently involved. The obligation in staging is to be certain that the hilus is free of tumor, utilizing CT scanning as the standard. If the hilus and lung parenchyma cannot be absolutely cleared on plain chest studies, it is obligatory to perform CT examination as the subsequent staging procedure. If the hilus is found to be involved by Hodgkin's disease, the radiation oncologist is obligated to treat the entire lung, adding significant morbidity to the patient. Uncommonly, following treatment, the mediastinal Hodgkin's lymph nodes, usually in the an-

TABLE 3-4.

Staging Classification, Hodgkin's Disease and Non-Hodgkin's Lymphoma*

Stage I	Involvement of a single lymph node region or single extralymphatic organ or site (I_E)
Stage II	Involvement of two or more lymph node regions on the same side of the diaphragm or localized involvement of an extralymphatic organ or site of one or more lymph node regions on the same side of the diaphragm (II_E)
Stage III	Involvement of lymph node regions on both sides of the diaphragm, which may be accompanied by localized involvement of extralymphatic organ or site (III_E), by involvement of the spleen (III_S), or both (III_{E+S})
Stage IV	Diffuse or disseminated involvement of one or more extralymphatic organs or tissues with or without associated lymph node enlargement. The reason for classifying the patient as stage IV is identified further by specifying sites such as the lung, bone, liver, brain, and so forth.

*Modified from American Joint Committee on Cancer, *Manual for Staging of Cancer*, ed 3. Philadelphia, J B Lippincott Co., 1988.

---

terior compartment, may undergo calcification. These calcifications are large, amorphous, and unique in appearance.

The NHL lesions less frequently involve the mediastinum and more often the lung parenchyma. Low-grade extranodal NHL may appear as a pulmonary infiltrate which persists, unchanged, for years. Staging of the NHLs is not as critical a process as with Hodgkin's disease, as the treatment more frequently is based on histology and organ sites of involvement than precise locations, unless radiation therapy is anticipated as the treatment modality. Pleural effusions can be noted with either Hodgkin's disease or the NHLs and are most frequently a manifestation of lymphatic obstruction by more central tumor as the effusions are virtually always negative for cells on cytologic evaluation.

Thymomas tend to be smaller lesions, particularly the solid tumors found in the patient population with myasthenia gravis. Thymic cysts have fluid-filled contents and, occasionally, rimlike calcifications within their walls.

The posterior mediastinum, generally included within the area subtended by the anterior vertebral bodies to the dorsal extent of the mediastinum, is the province of neurogenic tumors. A variety of ancillary findings may be noted, including enlargement of the neural foramen, a specific feature suggesting a neurofibroma. In young men, abnormalities of the vertebral body and thoracic cage will suggest that the posterior mediastinal lesion is a neurenteric cyst. Approximately 10% to 12% of neuroblastomas will involve the mediastinum as the primary site of disease, nearly always the posterior compartment. In these instances, the patient is older than with the usual neuroblastoma case (teenager vs. young child) and more frequently contains calcifications.

The middle mediastinum contains the heart, blood vessels, and lymphatics and the most frequent tumors within this compartment are related to those structures. The only primary lesion one should consider within the middle mediastinum is a bronchogenic cyst. These congenital lesions most frequently arise in the subcarinal region but may be found anywhere within the mediastinum and, occasionally, in the lung parenchyma. CT numbers should be of water density; however, if the lesion is infected, the CT numbers may be significantly greater than water density, suggesting a solid tumor. This is believed a function of the mucoid material or precipitation of crystalline material within the mass resulting from secondary infection.

Radiography

Even though some primary mediastinal tumors will initially be detected on plain chest x-rays, the CT scan is the primary means of both exploring the mediastinal compartments and detecting and defining the mediastinal tumors. The CT scan should be performed with 1 cm-interval sections, using contrast enhancement. To date, MR imaging has not shown significant advantage over CT scanning in the detection and definition of mediastinal tumors.

PRIMARY LUNG NEOPLASMS

This section concerns the solitary pulmonary nodule as discovered on the plain chest film, the diagnosis and staging of primary lung cancer, and an approach to pulmonary metastatic disease from an imaging vantage point.

The management of the pulmonary nodule or "coin lesion" is a complex radiographic problem which has been and continues to be a subject of considerable clinical and radiographic debate (Fig 3–1). The detection threshold for a mass lesion on a chest x-ray depends upon its location, contents, and marginal characteristics. A well-defined, smoothly marginated mass lesion in the lung can usually be seen on a properly exposed chest radiograph when its size exceeds 5 mm. This detection threshold can be reduced to 2 to 3 mm on CT scanning. Calcification within the solitary coin lesion virtually assures that the lesion is benign even though a "scar cancer" may engulf a preexisting calcified granuloma. The presence of calcification within a mass lesion has led to the suggestion that CT and the representative CT number could allow one to predict that a lesion was benign or malignant. So called "benign calcifications" tend to be central, homogeneous, or lam-

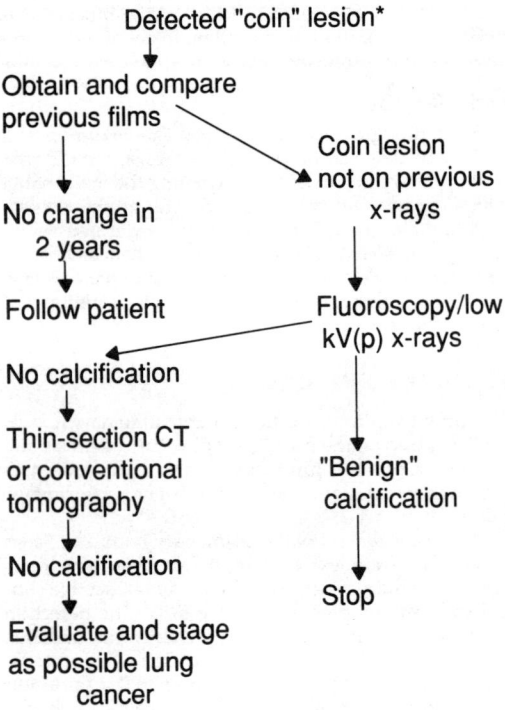

*Make certain "coin" lesion is not an artifact or skin lesion and is solitary.

FIG 3–1.
Radiographic evaluation of the solitary pulmonary nodule.

inated. The popcorn calcifications of hamartoma, although infrequently discovered, are diagnostic. Exceptions to the concept that calcifications identify benign lesions would be the presence of calcium or bone matrix within osteosarcoma or chondrosarcoma metastatic lesions to the chest. Siegelman et al. suggested in 1980 that a pulmonary nodule with a representative CT number of 164 or greater could safely be assumed to be benign. They presumed that diffuse calcification not visible on the plain film within these nodules led to the higher CT number. Practical difficulties in the application of this technique have limited its application. Ten institutions recently joined in an effort to evaluate 634 solitary pulmonary nodules, utilizing different CT units and a common phantom. They determined that a solitary pulmonary nodule can be reliably determined as benign if high attenuation values (no specific number was given) were found through at least 10% of the cross-sectional area of the nodule, and a well-defined margin was found. Solitary nodules examined by CT should be 2 cm or less in size. The plain film characteristics of benign calcifications within a pulmonary nodule are denseness, a central location, and a ringlike or "bull's eye" appearance.

It has been stated that a primary lung cancer must assume 1 cm in cross-sectional diameter to be visible on a routine chest x-ray. It is also estimated that radiologists "miss" between 30% and as high as 90% of primary lung cancers on the initial radiographic examination. The latter figure is derived from the experience of the recently completed National Lung Cancer Trial Programs, which showed that primary lung tumors in the periphery of the lung could be found in retrospect in nearly 90% of the cases.

Table 3–5 summarizes the four major types of primary lung cancers, their approximate frequency, and most common radiologic presenting characteristics. A great deal of overlap between these cancers occurs, but this table should form the basis of initial understanding

TABLE 3–5.
Lung Cancer: Pathologic Characteristics and Radiologic Features*

Histology	Approximate Frequency (%)	Parenchymal Abnormality	Features	5-Year Survival (%)
Squamous cell	35–50	Central, ill-defined mass, infiltrate or lobar collapse	Grows by direct invasion; obstructive pneumonia and collapse, cavitation, late metastasis	37
Small cell	20–30	Hilar mass	Grows by submucosal lymphatic extension; early hematogenous metastases, obstructive "pneumonia" and collapse	1
Adenocarcinoma	30–35	Peripheral, ill-defined nodule,	Early hematogenous metastases, rare	27

Large cell	5–15	mass, or infiltrate Peripheral large ill-defined mass	cavitation, scar carcinoma Very rapid growth, early lymphatic and hematogenous metastases, infrequent cavitation	27

*From Armstrong JD III, Bragg DG: Thoracic neoplasms, in *Oncologic Imaging*. New York, Pergamon Press, 1985, p 147. Reproduced by permission.

of the common radiologic features of these primary lung tumors.

As shown in Table 3–5, the four major categories of primary lung cancer include squamous (also referred to as epidermoid), adenocarcinoma (including bronchioloalveolar cell cancers), small cell anaplastic carcinomas (including oat cell cancers), and large cell anaplastic carcinomas (including giant cell and clear cell cancers). Until quite recently, squamous cell or epidermoid cancers represented the majority of all primary lung cancers; however, it now appears that adenocarcinoma has assumed that role. The reasons for this are controversial but include the increasing percentage of women with lung cancer, the broader use of electron microscopic classification, and other unknown factors. The model for lung cancer remains the squamous cell tumor. It is felt to arise from damaged and dysplastic bronchial epithelium, most often injured by cigarette smoking. The two primary lung cancers most closely associated with cigarette smoking are squamous cell cancers and small cell anaplastic cancers. Adenocarcinomas are felt to arise from the more peripheral elements of the lung, including the bronchial glands. Scar cancers are usually adenocarcinomas and often of the bronchioloalveolar type. The pathologist may find it quite difficult to distinguish a primary from a metastatic adenocarcinoma of the lung, a limitation that should be remembered by the radiologist in addressing this issue. Sputum cytology is most frequently positive with the more centrally located epidermoid carcinomas rather than the peripheral adenocarcinomas. Small cell anaplastic carcinomas include oat cell cancers as their most frequent tumor subtype. They were originally thought to be derived from neural ectoderm or the Kulchitsky cells. However, this is now a subject of considerable disagreement and debate. These tumors share a number of cytologic features with bronchial adenomas, an uncommon primary lung tumor which some consider to be malignant by behavior. Most of the bronchial adenomas (approximately 85%) are of carcinoid type and may be responsible for the carcinoid syndrome through serotonin byproducts not metabolized in the liver. Large cell anaplastic cancers are uncommon, representing between 15% and 20% of all primary lung tumors. The large cell cancers share many similarities radiographically and clinically with adenocarcinomas and may in fact be variants of that larger tumor category. Subtypes of this lesion include giant cell cancers and the clear cell lung cancer.

It is useful to consider the presenting radiologic characteristics of these different types of lung cancers to understand the more common radiographic features they exhibit. Epidermoid cancers and small cell carcinomas are principally central in origin in some 70% to 80% of the instances. Epidermoid cancers are the most common primary lung tumors to excavate, whether these lesions are primary or metastatic. The small cell anaplastic lesions rarely cavitate and often are manifest by hilar or mediastinal lymph node metastases with an occult primary lesion. In nearly 80% of the instances, small cell anaplastic lesions will have spread beyond the thorax at the time they initially present clinically or radiographically.

The two peripheral primary lung cancers are adenocarcinomas and large cell cancers. These lesions uncommonly cavitate and are usually initially detected by screening chest x-ray studies rather than sputum cytologic studies, in contrast to the epidermoid and small cell anaplastic cancers. Bronchioloalveolar cancers are the least aggressive of all primary lung tumors, at least when they present as a solitary peripheral coin lesion. Bronchioloalveolar cell cancers can also present with bilateral tumors or as an infiltrative, pneumonic process. In these latter instances, the prognosis is less favorable and the course more aggressive than with the solitary coin lesion mode of presentation.

The chest x-ray is usually adequate to establish the characteristics of the primary tumor; however, CT scanning or MR imaging is necessary to define the mediastinal extension of the tumor and determine the need for mediastinoscopy prior to definitive resection of the primary lung cancer. The role of CT is in detecting the enlarged mediastinal lymph node, which is greater than 1.5 or 2 cm and suspicious for involvement by metastatic tumor. These nodes must be further evaluated with either percutaneous biopsy or mediastinal exploration through mediastinotomy or mediastinoscopy.

There are no "pathognomonic" features on any imaging study of a primary lung cancer. Age can be used as a criteria to suggest the etiology of a solitary pulmonary nodule: a nodule in a child under the age of 12 is usually of congenital etiology; a nodule in a 20 or 30 year old is usually of an inflammatory nature; and a solitary lesion in a patient over the age of 50 who is a smoker is cancer until proved otherwise. Endobronchial lesions cause collapse of a segment or a lobe without the presence of an air bronchogram, as collateral air drift allows resorption of the air from the collapsed lung. Collapse of the left upper lobe in an older patient is almost always the result of a primary lung tumor which is endobronchial, and is usually a squamous cell cancer. The "S-sign of Golden" is the result of a central endobronchial lesion causing collapse of the right upper lobe without an air bronchogram and metastatic involvement of the hilus forming the medial portion of the "S" configuration.

Staging for primary lung cancer is an important process in which the radiologist plays a vital role. Lung cancer staging is performed according to the TNM system, a scheme now adopted worldwide. The TNM definitions are summarized in Tables 3–6 through 3–8. The T definition of the tumor can usually be determined by routine chest x-rays. None of our imaging techniques can enable us to accurately distinguish the margins of the tumor and host reaction in instances in which significant atelectasis or obstructive pneumonia, which frequently characterizes the central tumors, is present. The critical staging process and the most controversial one involves the determination of the N category. It is the determination of the node category and its histology that are the main determinants of survival and the primary elements in the therapeutic decision process. Stage I, non-oat cell cancer patients have a cumulative survival at 60 months of nearly 50%. This drops to approximately 25% for stage II patients, and nearly 10% for stage III patients. It is the primary role of imaging procedures to define those patients with abnormal, enlarged mediastinal lymph nodes. These lymph nodes should be biopsied to determine the cause for the enlargement, as the CT findings are nonspecific. Normal nodes tend to decrease in volume the further they are located from the hilus. Node size is obviously affected by nonneoplastic factors, such as contiguous infection. The radiologist should therefore detect the enlarged (nodes larger than 1.5 to 2.0 cm in short-axis CT measurement) to determine whether mediastinal biopsy is necessary prior to open thoracotomy. The presence or absence of hilar nodal involvement is less important in the staging process and generally of interest to the surgeon in helping to plan the appropriate resection strategy.

Radiography

Even though the chest x-ray study is flawed in terms of its detection efficiency, it remains the primary means of discovering primary lung cancer. The initial primary tumor staging (T category), usually can be adequately performed with plain chest films. CT scanning should be performed at 1-cm intervals from the angle of Louis to the subcarinal regions and then at intervals of every other centimeter from the thoracic inlet to include the adrenal glands, with contrast-material enhancement. Extrathoracic organ site exploration should be symptom-directed.

PULMONARY METASTATIC DISEASE

The radiographic patterns of pulmonary metastatic disease are summarized in Table 3–9. Sarcomas tend to spread to the lung in a hematogenous pattern, fa-

TABLE 3–6.
TNM Definitions: Primary Tumor (T)*

TX	Tumor proven by the presence of malignant cells in bronchopulmonary secretions but not visualized roentgenographically or bronchoscopically, or any tumor that cannot be assessed as in a retreatment staging
T0	No evidence of primary tumor
TIS	Carcinoma in situ
T1	A tumor that is 3.0 cm or less in greatest dimension, surrounded by lung or visceral pleura, and without evidence of invasion proximal to a lobar bronchus at bronchoscopy
T2	A tumor more than 3.0 cm in greatest dimension, or a tumor of any size that either invades the visceral pleura or has associated atelectasis or obstructive pneumonitis extending to the hilar region. At bronchoscopy, the proximal extent of demonstrable tumor must be within a lobar bronchus or at least 2.0 cm distal to the carina. Any associated atelectasis or obstructive pneumonitis must involve less than an entire lung.
T3	A tumor of any size with direct extension into the chest wall (including superior sulcus tumors), diaphragm, or the mediastinal pleura or pericardium without involving the heart, great vessels, trachea, esophagus, or vertebral body, or a tumor in the main bronchus within 2 cm of the carina without involving the carina.
T4	A tumor of any size with invasion of the mediastinum or involving heart, great vessels, trachea, esophagus, vertebral body, or car-

ina, or presence of malignant pleural effusion.

*From Mountain CF: A new international staging system for lung cancer. *Chest* 1986; 89(suppl)227S. Reproduced by permission.

TABLE 3–7.

TNM Definitions: Nodal Involvement (N)*

N0	No demonstrable metastasis to regional lymph nodes
N1	Metastasis to lymph nodes in the peribronchial or the ipsilateral hilar region, or both, including direct extension
N2	Metastasis to ipsilateral mediastinal lymph nodes and subcarinal lymph nodes
N3	Metastasis to contralateral mediastinal lymph nodes, contralateral hilar lymph nodes, ipsilateral or contralateral scalene, or supraclavicular lymph nodes

*From Mountain CF: A new international staging system for lung cancer. *Chest* 1986; 89(suppl) 227S. Reproduced by permission.

TABLE 3–8.

TNM Definitions: Distant Metastasis (M)*

M0	No (known) distant metastasis
M1	Distant metastasis present — specify site(s)

*From Mountain CF: A new international staging system for lung cancer. *Chest* 1986; 89(suppl) 227S. Reproduced by permission.

TABLE 3–9.
Pulmonary Metastatic Disease: Patterns and Probable Primary Sites*

Sarcomas	Nodular Pattern		Lymphangitic Pattern
	Epidermoid	Adenocarcinoma	"Always" adenocarcinoma (may occasionally be sarcomatous or epithelial)
	Head and neck	Colon	
		Prostate	
	Lung cancer	Lung	
	Head and neck	Kidney	

Male Patient	Female Patient
Lung primary (unilateral pattern)	Breast
Pancreas/stomach	Ovary
Prostate	

Cervix	Colon	
	Prostate	
	Lung	
	Kidney	
	Breast	
	Uterus	

*From Armstrong JD II, Bragg DG: Thoracic neoplasms, in *Oncologic Imaging*. New York, Pergamon Press, 1985, p 167. Reproduced by permission.

voring the lung base in size and number over the apex of the lung. Their margins are usually well defined as they tend not to incite a parenchymal reaction around the margins of the lesions. Squamous cell metastatic lesions have less well-defined margins and may undergo excavation, particularly at the lung apex. Adenocarcinomas have ill-defined margins, rarely excavate, and tend to involve the lung in a hematogenous pattern of distribution, similar to that described for the sarcomas. Lymphangitic tumor spread is a radiographic and pathologic expression of a metastatic tumor, almost always an adenocarcinoma which has usually reached the lung by hematogenous route. The adenocarcinoma then invades the lymphatics and causes lymphatic obstruction, producing a pattern which radiographically is quite similar to that of interstitial pulmonary edema from heart failure, with indistinct, prominent hilar structures and the visualization of septal lines (Kerley A, B, and C lines), pleural effusions, and occasionally, ill-defined, nodular parenchymal lesions. The Kerley lines are manifestations of thickened interlobular septa and represent engorged lymphatics/veins and, occasionally, fluid in the interlobular septa.

Surveillance of the lung in a patient with a primary tumor known to extend to the lung must be tailored to the behavior of the primary tumor. The selection of the appropriate imaging modality must depend upon the consequences of the detection of a pulmonary metastatic lesion. For example, in a child with an osteosarcoma prior to definitive treatment, the detection of a pulmonary lesion would drastically change the selection of a definitive treatment. In this instance, one can assume the higher false positive ratio of CT scanning of the thorax. The false positive findings may be as high as 50% in midwestern areas where the prevalence of histoplasmosis is significant.

Radiography

The radiographic evaluation of the patient suspected of metastatic pulmonary disease should be tailored to the known primary tumor. If the detection of metastatic pulmonary disease will significantly impact major treatment decisions, more aggressive radiologic staging can be justified, including CT scanning. In most instances, shallow oblique x-rays or film tomography is still useful in the detection of pulmonary metastatic lesions not visible on plain films, without accepting the increased challenge of pursuing the high yield of false positive, non-neoplastic lesions detected by more sophisticated imaging techniques such as CT.

BIBLIOGRAPHY

Aronberg DJ, Evans RG: Radiologic evaluation of the mediastinum. *Curr Probl Diagn Radiol* 1985; 15:6-35.

Armstrong JO II, Bragg DG: Thoracic neoplasms, in *Oncologic Imaging*. New York, Pergamon Press, 1985.

Bragg DG, Colby RB, Ward JH: New concepts in the non-Hodgkin lymphomas: Radiologic implications. *Radiology* 1986; 159:289-304.

Feigin DS, Siegelman SS, Theros EG, et al: Non-malignant lymphoid disorders of the chest. *AJR* 1977; 129:221-228.

Filderman AE, Shaw C, Matthay RA: Lung cancer. Part I: Etiology, pathology, natural history, manifestations and diagnostic techniques. *Invest Radiol* 1986; 21:80-90.

Griffiths H, Poster R, Robinson K: Solitary rib lesions. *Orthopedics* 1985; 8:802-811.

Heitzman ER: The role of computer tomography in the diagnosis and management of lung cancer. *Chest* 89(suppl):237S-241S.

Kennedy JL, Nathwani BN, Burke JS, et al: Pulmonary lymphomas and other pulmonary lymphoid lesions. *Cancer* 1985; 56:539-552.

McCloud TC, Woods BO, Carrington CB, et al: Diffuse pleural thickening in an asbestos-exposed population: Prevalence and causes. *AJR* 1985; 144:9-18.

Mountain CF: A new international staging system for lung cancer. *Chest* 1986; 89(suppl):225S-233S.

Muhm JR, Miller WE, Fontana RS, et al: Lung cancer detected during a screening program using 4-month chest radiographs. *Radiology* 1983; 148:609-615.

Seigelman SS, Khouri NF, Leo FP, et al: Solitary pulmonary nodules: CT assessment. *Radiology* 1986; 16:307-312.

Siegelman SS, Zerhouni EA, Leo FP, et al: CT of the solitary pulmonary nodule. *AJR* 1980; 135:1-13.

Wellner LJ, Putman CE: Imaging of occult pulmonary metastases: State-of-the-art. *CA* 1986; 36:48-58.

4 | Pulmonary Hypertension and Edema

Howard Mann, M.D.

KEY CONCEPTS

1. Pulmonary hypertension may occur when one or more of the following are increased: cardiac output; pulmonary venous pressure; and pulmonary vascular resistance.
2. In clinical practice, the most common causes of pulmonary hypertension are chronic hypoxia and left ventricular failure.
3. An analysis of the chest radiograph and radionuclide perfusion scan will aid in the differentiation between primary plexogenic arteriopathy, chronic thromboembolism, and pulmonary veno-occlusive disease.
4. Hydrostatic edema is distinguished from increased-permeability edema by the presence of cardiomegaly and signs of interstitial pulmonary edema.

PULMONARY HYPERTENSION

Definition and Terminology

The pulmonary circulation is a low-resistance, high-capacitance circuit, which is capable of accommodating increases in flow without a corresponding increase in pressure. This is achieved primarily by a combination of vascular distention and recruitment of nonperfused and/or hypoperfused microvessels. Pulmonary hypertension is present when pulmonary arterial pressure is inappropriately high for a given level of blood flow through the pulmonary circulation. By accepted definition, pulmonary hypertension is present when systolic pulmonary artery pressure is greater than 30 mm Hg. However, it should be remembered that pulmonary artery pressure increases with altitude as the amount of inspired oxygen decreases.

Pulmonary hypertension may occur as a primary phenomenon or secondary to pulmonary and/or cardiac disease. Secondary pulmonary hypertension is much more common, and a diagnosis of primary hypertension should only be made when objective testing fails to reveal a pulmonary or cardiac cause.

An understanding of the relevant pathophysiology underlying pulmonary hypertension will facilitate a rational approach to the differential diagnosis. An appreciation of factors that influence pulmonary vascular resistance is crucial, and these are incorporated in the following two formulas:

$$PVR = \frac{Ppa - Pla}{Q}. \tag{1}$$

PVR = pulmonary vascular resistance
Ppa = pulmonary artery pressure
Pla = left atrial pressure
Q = pulmonary blood flow.

Poiseuille's law (2)

$$R = P/Q = \frac{\Delta P \pi r^4}{8 \eta L}.$$

R = resistance
L = length
r = radius
η = viscosity
ΔP = pressure difference.

Thus, pulmonary artery pressure is influenced by cardiac output (Q), pulmonary venous pressure, blood viscosity, and the cross-sectional area of the vascular bed. A change in the length of pulmonary vessels is not a clinically significant factor. Established causes of pulmonary hypertension will affect one or a combination of these parameters as discussed later.

Increased Cardiac Output

An increase in blood flow through the lungs will be associated with an increase in pulmonary artery pressures, leading to a decrease in vascular resistance as distention and recruitment of intrapulmonary vessels occur. Large and persistent increases in flow, such as left-to-right shunts through intracardiac septal defects, will result in secondary, irreversible changes in the arterial tree, consisting primarily of muscularization of large pulmonary arteries and extension of muscle into smaller, more peripheral arteries (neomuscularization). The resultant increase in pulmonary vascular resistance contributes further to pulmonary hypertension.

Increased Pulmonary Venous Pressure

Increased left atrial/pulmonary venous pressure is a common cause of pulmonary hypertension in clinical practice. An elevated pulmonary artery pressure serves to maintain a necessary gradient for flow across the pulmonary vascular bed. Causes in this category include left ventricular (congestive) failure, mitral stenosis, and congenital stenosis of the pulmonary veins.

Increased Pulmonary Vascular Resistance

In this category, the clinically important factors that contribute to a decreased effective radius of the vascular bed are as follows.

Decreased Luminal Diameter.—Morphologic.— For example, smooth muscle hypertrophy due to chronic hypoxia, occlusion due to perivascular fibrosis/granuloma formation, narrowing due to intimal hyperplasia/fibrosis.

Vasoconstriction.—Acute hypoxia.

Luminal Vascular Obstruction.—Pulmonary embolism, tumor embolism, and in situ thrombosis (e.g., hemoglobin SS sickle-cell disease).

Loss of Vessels.—Pulmonary resection, emphysema.

Of course, in many conditions a combination of these factors will contribute to increased vascular resistance.

Radiography of Pulmonary Hypertension

The primary radiographic sign of pulmonary hypertension is dilatation of pulmonary artery shadows on the chest radiograph. In particular, there is dilatation of the main pulmonary artery, producing a convexity beneath the aortic knob, and dilatation of the central left and right pulmonary arteries.

Elevated arterial pressure leads to increased caliber of intrapulmonary artery shadows as a result of increased transmural pressures. For example, the diameter of the upper lobe anterior segmental artery will be greater than the diameter of the companion anterior segmental bronchus, when visible on the frontal projection. On the frontal, erect radiograph, the size of vessels in the upper lung zones may approach that in the lower lung zones. This appearance should not be considered a sign of increased flow per se, a common misinterpretation. Chronic hypertension leads to structural remodeling involving vessel walls and a corresponding reduction in cross-sectional area and increased resistance. This may manifest as "pruning" on the chest radiograph, with a fairly abrupt decrease in caliber between the large, dilated central arteries and the more peripheral vascular segments. This may occur in diverse causes of pulmonary hypertension such as high-flow states and chronic hypoxia. Enlargement of the right ventricle and right atrium may be seen.

Once these features are identified, radiographic signs of specific pulmonary and/or cardiac disorders should be evaluated. These are described in the relevant sections of this handbook.

Diagnostic Approach to Pulmonary Hypertension

Step 1: History and Physical Examination

This will readily reveal the most common causes of secondary pulmonary hypertension—chronic hypoxia due to chronic lung disease and congestive heart failure (left ventricular failure). In addition, the following disorders should be excluded.

Connective Tissue Disorders.—Scleroderma and CREST syndrome, systemic lupus erythematosus, mixed connective tissue disease, and rheumatoid arthritis.

Hepatic Disease.—In this situation, right-to-left intrapulmonary shunting at the microvascular level is postulated to be the cause of secondary pulmonary hypertension.

Drug Ingestion.—Drugs that have been implicated include aminorex, phenformin, and possibly oral contraceptives. Drug abusers may inject the dissolved contents of crushed pills that include talc or microcrystalline cellulose, leading to an obliterative perivascular granulomatous reaction.

Hemoglobinopathies.—Hemoglobin SS and SC sickle-cell disease. In situ thrombosis leads to increased vascular resistance.

Metastatic Malignancy.—Tumor embolism to the pulmonary microcirculation may present as pulmonary hypertension. Carcinomas of the breast, lung, stomach, pancreas, prostate, and choriocarcinoma are those most commonly reported.

Step 2: Exclude Left-to-Right Shunt and Eisenmenger's Physiology

Increased pulmonary blood flow due to left-to-right intracardiac shunts is an important cause of pulmonary hypertension in the pediatric age group. In the adult, an unsuspected atrial septal defect is most prevalent. Patients may present with signs and symptoms of pulmonary hypertension. If pulmonary pressures are sufficiently high, flow reversal with a right-to-left shunt may occur; this is termed Eisenmenger's physiology. There are many invasive and noninvasive tests that may be used to exclude this as a cause:

Cardiac Catheterization and Angiography.—Intracardiac, pulmonary artery and wedge pressures may be obtained. A step-up in blood oxygen saturation may be obtained during passage of the catheter through the right side of the heart. Coincident valvular abnormalities may be identified. In the face of elevated pulmonary artery pressures and a normal wedge pressure, pulmonary veno-occlusive disease should be suspected.

Radionuclide Ventriculography.—This may establish the presence of a right-to-left shunt through a patent foramen ovale in the presence of Eisenmenger's physiology. In addition, global function of the cardiac chambers may be studied in a dynamic mode.

Echocardiography.—This is an excellent means of evaluating cardiac/valvular function. Two-dimensional ultrasound will demonstrate interatrial/interventricular septal defects. This may be combined with Doppler-derived information concerning intracardiac blood flow, and contrast echocardiography to evaluate shunting across the interatrial septum. Left atrial myxomas may be identified.

Step 3: Further Evaluation of Apparent Primary Pulmonary Hypertension

Once pulmonary venous hypertension and left-to-right shunting are excluded as causes, attention should be directed to increased vascular resistance. Other than increased resistance due to chronic hypoxia, three disorders may present as "primary" hypertension: (1) primary plexogenic arteriopathy; (2) chronic pulmonary thromboembolism; and (3) pulmonary veno-occlusive disease.

Primary Plexogenic Arteriopathy.—This disorder affects mainly young women and children. Patients typically present with dyspnea on exertion as a main complaint. The prognosis is dismal, with an average survival of only several years. Pathologically, there is vascular occlusion characterized by an increased thickness of the muscular coat of normally muscular arteries, intimal hyperplasia, and the formation of plexiform lesions of proliferating intimal and endothelial cells. In some patients, thrombi are noted in the pulmonary microvasculature, probably representing in situ thrombosis. Whether these patients may benefit from chronic anticoagulation is uncertain.

Chronic Pulmonary Thromboembolism.—This may occur as a result of recurrent episodes of pulmonary embolism. Rarely, it may represent an episode of unresolved acute pulmonary embolism, with large remnant clot in the central pulmonary arteries. In individual cases, it may be difficult to distinguish between embolism and in situ thrombosis. Many investigators believe that chronic pulmonary hypertension results in endothelial damage and a procoagulant environment, predisposing to in situ thrombosis. Patients in this group tend to be older and may or may not have a history of recurrent deep vein thrombosis and episodes of dyspnea and chest pain. Pathologically, there may be thrombi of varying age, eccentric intimal fibrosis and intraluminal fibrous septa/webs.

Pulmonary Veno-occlusive Disease.— This disorder may produce signs and symptoms indistinguishable from pulmonary venous hypertension due to left ventricular failure. In its typical form, there is occlusion of small pulmonary veins. Catheterization reveals elevated pulmonary artery pressures with a normal or low wedge pressure. Pathologically, there is predominantly fibrointimal occlusion of vascular lumens with myxoid, paucicellular connective tissue. Recanalization with formation of intraluminal fibrous septa is common, raising the possibility of in situ thrombosis as a predisposing pathophysiologic event.

This condition is usually idiopathic, but has been described as a complication of cytotoxic chemotherapy. Viral infections have been implicated as a cause. In adults, men are affected more often than women, unlike the female predominance in primary plexogenic arteriopathy.

The differentiation between these three disorders may be difficult, particularly when the chest radiograph reveals only dilated pulmonary arteries. However, an evaluation of the chest radiograph along with a perfusion scan will facilitate the diagnostic work-up when the patterns shown in Table 4–1 are found.

The distinction between plexogenic arteriopathy and proximal thromboembolism may be important as surgical thromboembolectomy in suitable patients in the latter group may be feasible.

A Guide to Imaging Procedures in the Evaluation of Pulmonary Hypertension

Many imaging modalities other than chest radiographs may be utilized during the evaluation of a patient with pulmonary hypertension. Obviously, this reflects the large number of possible etiologies, from common to rare disorders. The following modalities have been demonstrated to have specific diagnostic efficacy.

Pulmonary Angiography.— Acute and chronic pulmonary thromboembolism; arteriovenous malformations; pulmonary vein stenosis (intrinsic and extrinsic);

TABLE 4–1.
Differentiation of Apparent Primary Pulmonary Hypertension

Disorder	Radiograph	Perfusion Scan
Primary plexogenic arteriopathy	No parenchymal/pleural process	Normal
Chronic (proximal) pulmonary embolism	No parenchymal/pleural process	Segmental/subsegmental defects
Pulmonary veno-occlusive disease	Interstitial edema/effusions	Inhomogeneous perfusion/nonsegmental defects

Computed Tomography.—Chronic, proximal pulmonary thromboembolism; and idiopathic/granulomatous fibrosing mediastinitis.

Cardiac Ultrasound.—Left-to-right shunt lesions; atrial myxoma; and valvular disease.

Magnetic Resonance Imaging.—Left-to-right shunts due to septal defects; atrial myxoma; chronic pulmonary thromboembolism.

Radionuclide Studies.—Pulmonary embolism (PE)/perfusion abnormalities; intracardiac shunts; and cardiac chamber size/function.

PULMONARY EDEMA

Pulmonary edema represents abnormal accumulation of extravascular water in the lung. In practical terms, this occurs when the rate of fluid filtration from the vascular compartment exceeds the rate of clearance from the interstitial compartment of the lung. After a certain amount of fluid has accumulated within the interstitial compartment, alveolar flooding occurs. While edema confined to the interstitial compartment may not significantly affect gas-exchange across the alveolar-capillary barrier, alveolar edema is always clinically significant. Thus, the recognition of interstitial edema on a chest radiograph will facilitate earlier, appropriate treatment.

Pathophysiology of Pulmonary Edema

An appreciation of the forces that govern fluid movement across the endothelial barrier is a useful starting point when considering clinical conditions that may cause pulmonary edema. The classic Starling equation relates the forces as follows:

$$\dot{Q}f = Kf\left[(Pmv - Ppmv) - \sigma(\pi mv - \pi pmv)\right] \quad (3)$$

where K_f is the filtration coefficient, describing the permeability characteristics of the endothelial barrier for water; Pmv and $Ppmv$ are the hydrostatic pressures in the microvascular and perimicrovascular interstitial spaces, respectively; πmv and πpmv are the colloid osmotic (oncotic) pressures in the plasma and interstitial spaces; and σ is the colloid reflection coefficient, that defines the effectiveness of the barrier in preventing the movement of colloid, compared with the flow of water.

In the normal person, there is normally a net outward filtration of fluid from the microvascular to the perimicrovascular spaces, estimated at 10 to 20 ml/hr in adults. This amount is easily removed to the thoracic systemic veins by the pulmonary lymphatics.

Two major categories of pulmonary edema are encountered in clinical practice: hydrostatic and increased-permeability edema. Hydrostatic edema results when elevated microvascular pressures are responsible for increased fluid filtration. The common causes in this instance are congestive heart failure (pulmonary venous hypertension) and overhydration edema, usually in association with renal failure and/or iatrogenic fluid overload. Increased-permeability edema, sometimes called noncardiogenic edema, results when there is a loss of the integrity of the microvascular barrier with respect to liquid and protein flow. The filtration coefficient increases while the protein reflection coefficient decreases. In this situation, even small increases in microvascular pressures will result in disproportionate accumulation of extravascular fluid. The edema fluid recovered in this situation typically contains a high protein concentration, usually above 70% of the plasma level. Important causes of this form of edema in clinical practice are aspiration of gastric acid, sepsis (pulmonary infection and septicemia), and hypotensive shock and embolism of toxic substances, such as fat embolism. Increased-permeability edema is the initial and predominant radiographic feature in acute lung injury as-

Sequence of Fluid Accumulation in the Lung

An orderly sequence of fluid accumulation occurs in the formation of pulmonary edema, particularly evident with hydrostatic edema when fluid accumulation is relatively slow. Filtered fluid initially enters the perimicrovascular, septal interstitial space (particularly the "thick" portion of the interalveolar septum) and then flows passively along a hydraulic pressure gradient to the terminal lymphatics adjacent to the bronchoarterial bundles in the terminal respiratory unit, and the lymphatics in the interlobular septa. In addition, there is a hydraulic pressure gradient from the peripheral peribronchovascular interstitium to the central, hilar peribronchovascular compartment. The thickness of these peribronchovascular fluid cuffs is related to lung volumes; increased volumes are associated with increased negative interstitial pressure, facilitating fluid accumulation. Thus, a central movement of edema fluid results, keeping the gas-exchanging portions of the lungs "dry." When a critical volume is reached, alveolar edema forms in individual alveoli or groups of alveoli on an all-or-nothing basis. The exact site of fluid entry into the alveoli is still a matter of debate, but may be through the terminal airway epithelium at the bronchoalveolar junction.

Radiography of Pulmonary Edema

Interstitial edema in congestive heart failure is generally evident radiographically when left atrial pressure exceeds 18 to 20 mm Hg. The following features may be seen:

1. Peribronchial fluid cuffs. These are initially present in the hilar regions, around proximal segmental/subsegmental bronchi. Care should be taken not to confuse this sign with bronchial wall thickening due to

other disorders such as asthma and chronic bronchitis. Comparison should be made with previous radiographs if these are available.

2. Septal lines. These thin lines represent fluid accumulation within interlobular septa. These are popularly referred to as Kerley's lines, named for their characteristic appearance and location on the radiograph as illustrated in Figure 4–1. Septal lines are also seen on the lateral projection, particularly in the retrosternal area.

3. Subpleural edema. This appears as apparent thickening of the interlobar fissures, often simulating pleural fluid within the fissures. In this situation, fluid is present within the subpleural connective tissue compartment, which is anatomically continuous with the interstitial compartment in the interlobular septa.

4. Perivascular interstitial edema. This renders the margins of pulmonary vessels indistinct. This may be most evident in the dependent portion of the lung where fluid accumulation tends to be greatest, at least in hydrostatic edema.

The accumulation of interstitial edema in congestive heart failure is associated with a reduction of lung compliance and vital capacity. Thus, decreasing lung volumes is a useful sign of increasing extravascular lung water.

Alveolar edema occurs when left atrial pressure exceeds 20 to 25 mm Hg, and is influenced by the plasma protein concentration. Hypoalbuminemia will promote edema formation at lower microvascular pressures. Alveolar edema has all the usual features of airspace consolidation: poor margination, representing the uneven involvement and superimposition of opacified pulmonary lobules; coalescing opacities; nonsegmental distribution; and air bronchograms. In hydrostatic edema, alveolar fluid accumulates predominantly in the dependent lung regions. This gravitational effect on microvascular pressures promoting fluid filtration is most evident when the patient is placed in a decubitus po-

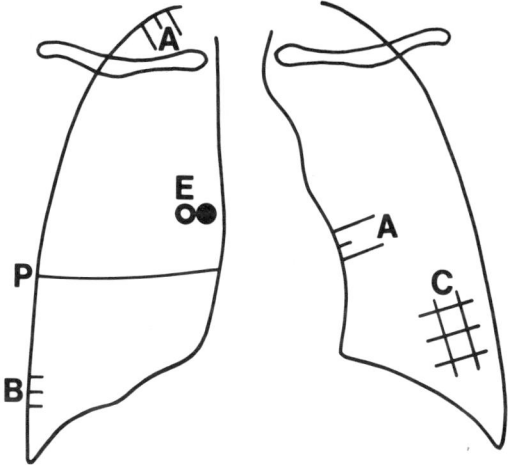

FIG 4–1.
Diagrammatic representation of interstitial edema. (*A* = Kerley A line; *B* = Kerley B line; *C* = Kerley C line; *E* = peribronchial fluid cuff; *P* = subpleural edema.)

sition, when the fluid will "shift" to the dependent lung.

Radiographic Differentiation Between Hydrostatic and Increased-Permeability Pulmonary Edema

The appearance of the chest radiograph may aid in the distinction between the three major categories of edema: cardiogenic [congestive heart failure (CHF)]; overhydration/renal; and increased-permeability edema. The following features should be analyzed on the frontal radiograph: heart size; width of the vascular pedicle; size of the azygous vein; the presence of septal lines/peribronchial fluid cuffs; pleural effusions; soft tissue

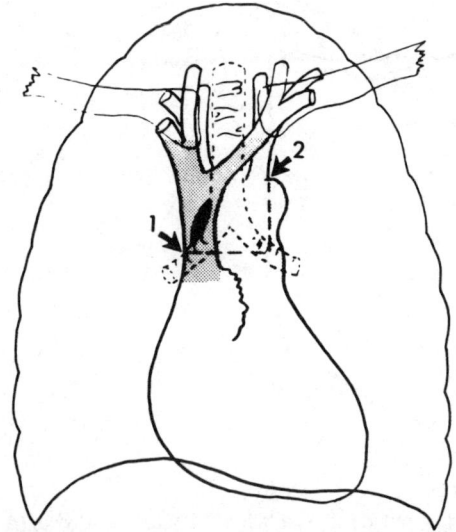

FIG 4–2.
Landmarks of the vascular pedicle. *1* = point where superior vena cava crosses right main stem bronchus; *2* = origin of left subclavian artery. (Modified from Milne ENC, Pistolesi M, Miniati M, et al: Vascular pedicle of the heart and the vena azygous. *Radiology* 1984; 152:1–8.)

thickness (edema) along the lateral chest wall; and the distribution of alveolar edema.

Heart Size

Cardiomegaly is generally present in CHF. The heart may also be enlarged when there is marked expansion of total blood volume owing to iatrogenic fluid overload and/or renal failure.

The Vascular Pedicle

This term refers to the dimensions of the large systemic vessels in the superior mediastinum, as illustrated in Figure 4–2.

The width of the vascular pedicle correlates well with total blood volume and is increased in overhydration edema. Although mean values for the width of the pedicle have been proposed, serial assessment in relation to previous radiographs is most useful. The width may also be increased in CHF associated with renal fluid retention, but generally not to the extent commonly seen in iatrogenic fluid overload/chronic renal failure.

Azygous Vein

The size of the azygous vein on the frontal radiograph is influenced by right atrial pressure and will indirectly reflect changes in total blood volume. As with the width of the vascular pedicle, serial assessment of its size on comparable radiographs will be useful. Allowances should be made for other factors that influence its size such as patient position (supine vs. erect), radiographic magnification (posteroanterior vs. anteroposterior) technique, body size, and other causes of elevated right atrial pressure.

Septal Lines

Septal lines and other signs of interstitial edema such as peribronchial fluid cuffs/subpleural edema are prevalent in CHF, and to a lesser extent in overhydration edema. Fluid accumulation tends to be relatively rapid in increased-permeability edema, which typically manifests with diffuse alveolar edema in the absence of conventional signs of interstitial edema.

Pleural Effusion

This is common in CHF and overhydration, but may be seen in "pure" increased-permeability edema. Pleural fluid represents transudation of fluid from the visceral pleural surface into the pleural space, and is cleared by subpleural lymphatics on the parietal pleural side. This may occur when hydrostatic pressure in small subvisceral pulmonary veins increases in pulmonary venous hypertension. Pleural fluid also represents bulk movement of pulmonary edema fluid into the pleural space, keeping the lung parenchyma "dry." **It is important to remember that pleural effusions in congestive heart failure correlate with elevated left, but not right, atrial pressure.**

Chest Wall Soft Tissue Edema

Serial assessment of the thickness of the soft tissues adjacent to the lateral rib margins will complement physical examination, urinalysis, and daily measurements of body weight in the evaluation of total body water.

Distribution of Alveolar Edema

The distribution of hydrostatic edema is influenced by gravitational effects on microvascular pressures. Fluid filtration in this instance tends to be greatest in the dependent regions of the lung. In increased-permeability edema, the distribution of edema primarily reflects local/regional disruption of the alveolar-capillary barrier. This is reflected in the prevalence and distribution of air bronchograms, which are more common in increased-permeability edema.

The differentiation between cardiogenic (hydrostatic) and increased-permeability edema is summarized in Table 4–2.

TABLE 4–2.
Useful Differential Factors in Cardiogenic and Increased-Permeability Edema

Cardiogenic Edema	Increased-Permeability Edema
Enlarged heart	Normal heart size
Septal lines common	Septal lines uncommon
Air bronchograms uncommon	Air bronchograms common

SELECTED REFERENCES

Heitzman ER: *The Lung. Radiologic-Pathologic Correlations.* St Louis, C V Mosby Co, 1984, pp 79-92.

Koerner SK: Pulmonary hypertension: Etiology and clinical evaluation. *J Thorac Imaging* 1988; 3(1):25.

Milne ENC, Pistolesi M, Miniati M, et al: Radiologic distinction of cardiogenic and noncardiogenic edema. *AJR* 1985; 144:879.

Milne ENC, Pistolesi M, Miniati M, et al: Vascular pedicle of the heart and the vena azygous. *Radiology* 1984; 152:1.

Powe JE, Palevsky HI, McCarthy KE, et al: Pulmonary arterial hypertension: Value of perfusion scintigraphy. *Radiology* 1987; 164:727.

Rich S, Dantzker D, Ayers S, et al: Primary pulmonary hypertension. *Ann Intern Med* 1987; 107:216.

Rich S, Levitsky S, Brundage BH: Pulmonary hypertension from chronic pulmonary thromboembolism *Ann Intern Med* 1988; 108:425.

Rich S, Pietra GG, Kieras K, et al: Primary pulmonary hypertension: Radiographic and scintigraphic patterns of histologic subtypes. *Ann Intern Med* 1986; 105:499.

Rounds S, Hill NS: Pulmonary hypertensive diseases. *Chest* 1984; 85:397.

Smith RC, Mann H, Greenspan RH, et al: Radiographic differentiation between different etiologies of pulmonary edema. *Invest Radiol* 1987; 22:859.

Staub NC: Pathophysiology of pulmonary edema, in Staub NC, Taylor AE (eds): *Edema.* New York, Raven Press, 1984, pp 719-746.

Wagenvoort CA, Wagenvoort N, Takahashi T: Pulmonary veno-occlusive disease. *Hum Pathol* 1985; 16:1033.

5

Pulmonary Thromboembolism

Howard Mann, M.D.

KEY CONCEPTS

1. Venous thrombosis is the primary event in pulmonary embolism (PE).
2. A normal chest radiograph does not exclude the diagnosis of PE.
3. A normal radionuclide perfusion scan excludes clinically significant PE.
4. A pretest estimate of the probability of PE should be combined with the result of a ventilation/perfusion scan to yield a posttest probability of PE. The latter should guide management decisions.
5. Pulmonary tumor embolism may be associated with dyspnea, hypoxemia, and a normal chest radiograph.
6. Fat embolism presents with diffuse consolidation owing to diffuse alveolar damage.
7. Septic embolism presents with bilateral nodules which may cavitate.

ACUTE PULMONARY EMBOLISM

Pulmonary embolism (PE) is a major cause of morbidity and mortality in the United States, with an estimated 600,000 cases occurring annually. Autopsy studies have shown that a relatively large number of cases are not diagnosed before death, as the symptoms and signs of PE are nonspecific, and PE occurs commonly in hospitalized patients with other serious medical and/or surgical disorders. In addition, PE may be responsible for substantial morbidity and mortality in patients with no preexisting cardiopulmonary disease. This group includes hospitalized patients immobilized for extended periods of time and patients undergoing surgical procedures known to be associated with a definite risk of PE (e.g., the elderly patient with a hip fracture admitted for hip arthroplasty). When PE is diagnosed and appropriately treated, the mortality rate of approximately 30% in the untreated group is significantly reduced, thus providing incentive for prompt diagnosis whenever a clinical situation is associated with a high likelihood of PE. However, the treatment and prophylaxis of thromboembolism with anticoagulants are associated with a definite risk of hemorrhagic complications; thus the diagnosis has to be established with a high degree of certainty before a commitment to anticoagulation is made.

Pathophysiology

Venous thrombosis is the primary etiologic event that may be complicated by PE. Venous thrombosis may be clinically silent or may be misdiagnosed; as the symptoms and signs of thrombosis are nonspecific. The first sign of venous thrombosis may be the occurrence of PE. The vast majority of emboli derive from the deep venous system of the lower extremities and pelvis. From a clinical and statistical standpoint, thrombosis involving the proximal veins of the leg and pelvis (popliteal, femoral, and iliac) appears to be most relevant, and emboli may arise from multiple sites. It is uncertain how often embolism from thrombosis confined to the deep veins of the lower leg (calf) or small veins of the pelvis, such as periprostatic or periuterine veins, is clinically significant. Pulmonary emboli may also arise from thrombus in the inferior vena cava (IVC), central veins such as the superior vena cava and innominate veins, and the right atrium. Predisposing factors to venous thrombosis are immobilization, obesity, pregnancy, congestive heart failure, coagulopathies, direct trauma, tumor compression of large veins, and use of drugs such as oral contraceptives.

Pulmonary embolism may or may not be associated with pulmonary infarction. It is established fact that embolism without infarction is much more common than embolism with infarction; true infarction (tissue necrosis) probably occurs in less than 1% of patients with acute PE. When a variable portion of the pulmonary arterial tree is occluded by emboli, collateral circulation from the bronchial arterial tree through precapillary bronchopulmonary anastamoses is sufficient to prevent ischemic necrosis. Indeed, acute and complete occlusion of a main left or right pulmonary artery in a normal subject will not be associated with any untoward acute effects. However, the prevalence of infarction is increased in patients with congestive heart failure, presumably as a result of a deleterious efect of elevated pulmonary venous pressures and decreased cardiac output on blood flow through bronchopulmonary anastomotic channels.

Approximately 75% of emboli lodge in the lower lungs, corresponding to the regional distribution of pulmonary blood flow. Pulmonary embolism typically affects multiple vessels in both lungs; thus, multiple infarcts are at least twice as common as single infarcts when the lungs are evaluated pathologically.

Clinical Diagnosis

Because the symptoms and signs of PE are nonspecific, patients may present with chest pain, dyspnea, tachypnea, hypotension, hypoxia, cardiac arrhythmias, and hemoptysis—findings that may be seen in various combinations in many other conditions such as myocardial infarction, pneumonia, pericarditis, aortic dissection, and pneumothorax. In addition, the clinical diagnosis of deep venous thrombosis (DVT) in the lower leg is similarly associated with high false negative and false positive rates. Thus, more objective imaging techniques play a crucial role in the diagnosis of PE.

A summary of imaging and other diagnostic procedures that may be utilized is presented in Table 5–1. Those that have a well-established role are emphasized, and will be elaborated upon subsequently.

Lower Limb Venography

The documentation of DVT as an indication for anticoagulation will obviate the need for pulmonary angiography, and this procedure has been advocated as the initial test in this clinical situation. However, as with pulmonary angiography, venography exposes the patient to the risks associated with contrast medium administration, and the procedure itself will cause DVT in a small number of patients. Lower extremity venography frequently does not result in adequate visualization of the common iliac veins and IVC. These vessels may be studied when pulmonary angiography is performed from the femoral route. Thus, pulmonary angiography should be considered the study of choice when a procedure utilizing radiographic contrast material is to be performed in a patient with suspected PE. If contrast venography is performed and results in a normal study, PE is not excluded, as studies have reported normal venograms in the presence of PE in up to 30% of patients. If a pulmonary angiogram is negative for PE in spite of a high index of suspicion on the basis of clinical findings and the result of a ventilation-perfusion scan, lower-limb venography should be considered. This relates to the fact that false negative results have been described with pulmonary angiography, although this is uncommon.

Chest Radiography

Chest radiographic findings in PE are protean but unfortunately nonspecific. The following may be seen alone or in varying combinations: focal parenchymal opacity/opacities, atelectasis, effusion, diaphragmatic elevation, regional oligemia, distended proximal pulmonary artery, enlargement of the right side of the heart, and, importantly, a normal chest radiograph.

TABLE 5–1.
Imaging Modalities and Procedures Used in Diagnosis of Deep Vein Thrombosis and Pulmonary Embolism

Deep Vein Thrombosis	Pulmonary Embolism
Lower limb venography*	Chest radiography*
Duplex sonography*	Ventilation/perfusion scan*
Impedance plethysmography	Pulmonary angiography*
Radionuclide venography	

*Denotes well-established role in diagnosis of pulmonary embolism.

Parenchymal abnormalities relate to the underlying pathophysiology which may be grouped as follows:

1. PE without infarction. Following obstruction of a pulmonary artery, the distal capillary bed may be perfused from adjacent patent microvessels. The capillaries will become congested, but remain intact. The occluded vessel will be recanalized over time. If the area of ischemia is sufficiently large, capillary disruption will occur, and blood flow under systemic pressure through bronchopulmonary anastamoses will result in a localized zone of edema and hemorrhage. Tissue necrosis does not occur.
2. PE with infarction. Rarely, particularly in the presence of pulmonary venous hypertension, collateral blood flow is insufficient to prevent the onset of true pale infarction. This area of infarction is invariably surrounded by a viable but hemorrhagic zone of variable size.

Pulmonary Embolism Without Infarction. — The chest radiograph may be normal or reveal regional oligemia—the so-called Westermark's sign. Of all the aforementioned radiographic findings, regional oligemia in association with dilated proximal pulmonary arteries, when a new finding, is most suggestive of PE. Unfortunately, this sign occurs infrequently. A more common finding is localized consolidation representing pulmonary hemorrhage, which may resolve in a short period of time.

Pulmonary Embolism With Infarction. — In this situation, a zone of atelectasis and pulmonary hemorrhage frequently surrounds and initially obscures an associated area of infarcted, necrotic lung. As the hemorrhage begins to resolve, a nonsegmental, focal opacity may become apparent—a Hampton's hump. This is classically situated adjacent to a pleural surface, but is infrequently perfectly wedge-shaped or well marginated, as it represents a random combination of infarcted and viable pulmonary lobules. With time, the infarcted area may shrink until only a small irregular or linear opacity remains.

A chest radiograph should always be obtained when PE is suspected:

1. To rule out other causes. The chest radiograph may reveal an unsuspected, alternative cause for the patient's symptoms such as pulmonary edema in association with myocardial infarction, or a pneumothorax.
2. To assess the presence or absence of the aforementioned radiographic signs, but not to exclude the possibility of PE on the basis of a normal radiograph.
3. To aid in the interpretation of ventilation/perfusion (V/Q) scans.

The accuracy of the chest radiograph alone in the diagnosis of PE has been studied: the average sensitivity was 33% (range, 0.52 to 0.08) and the average specificity was 59% (range, 0.31 to 0.80). Thus, additional objective diagnostic tests are mandatory.

Ventilation/Perfusion Scanning

This procedure should be performed as the next imaging test in the diagnostic approach to suspected PE. Traditionally, the perfusion scan has been the mainstay of this scintigraphic procedure, but the addition of a ventilation scan improves its specificity, permitting a more meaningful estimate of the likelihood of PE in the individual patient.

Pulmonary embolism results in perfusion defects with ventilation/perfusion mismatch—areas of lung that are not perfused but normally ventilated. The scintigraphic hallmark of pulmonary embolism is the presence of multiple, bilateral segmental perfusion defects with normal ventilation of these areas. Ventilation/perfusion scans are interpreted in conjunction with a concurrently obtained chest radiograph in order to correlate perfusion defects with opacities that may be present on the radiograph. It is presumed that these opacities represent areas of lung that are not normally ventilated, resulting in corresponding perfusion defects due to hypoxic vasoconstriction. Such matched perfusion defects mitigate against a diagnosis of PE. In general, the interpretation of the V/Q scan is reported as a probabilistic estimate of the likelihood of pulmonary embolism: high ($\geq$90%), low ($\leq$10%), and intermediate. The various combinations of findings on the perfusion scan, ventilation scan, and chest radiograph with corresponding estimates of the likelihood of PE are listed in Table 5–2.

It is very important to integrate the probabilistic estimate of PE based on these diagnostic criteria with a prior clinical estimate of the likelihood of PE in each individual patient. This approach, a clinical application of Baye's theorem, which takes into account the sensitivity and specificity of a test along with a pretest probability estimate, will result in a posttest probability of PE, which should then guide patient management and the decision to obtain a pulmonary angiogram. In general, a scan pattern resulting in an intermediate probability of PE may not substantially alter the prescan, clinical estimate of the likelihood of PE, and should be followed by the performance of a pulmonary angiogram in most patients. In addition, patients at high risk for hemorrhagic complications of anticoagulation should undergo angiography even when a high probability scan pattern is obtained. Other indications for pulmonary angiography are detailed in the suggested diagnostic strategy outlined below.

In summary, a V/Q scan should always be obtained for the following reasons:

1. A normal perfusion scan excludes PE.
2. High and low probability scan patterns, evaluated in conjunction with a prior clinical estimate of the likelihood of PE, may obviate the need for pulmonary angiography.

TABLE 5–2.

Diagnostic Criteria for V/Q Scan Interpretation*

Probability of PE	Diagnostic Reference Criteria
0	Normal perfusion
Low	Small Q defects regardless of number, V or CXR findings
	Q defects substantially smaller than CXR defect (V irrelevant)
	V-Q match in <50% one lung or <75% of one lung zone. CXR normal or nearly normal
	Single moderate Q with normal CXR
	Nonsegmental Q defects
Intermediate	Abnormality not defined by either "high" or "low" probability criteria
High	Two or more large Q. V and CXR normal
	Two or more large Q in which Q is much larger than either matching V or CXR
	Two or more moderate Q and one large Q. V and CXR normal
	Four or more moderate Q. V and CXR normal

*"Small" is a lesion involving <25% of the area of a pulmonary segment, "moderate" is equivalent to 25% to 75% of a segment, and "large" means more than 75% of a segment. Chest x-ray (CXR) defect indicates radiographic opacity in the region related to the Q and V lesion. When CXR is "normal," this alludes to CXR appearance in the region of the V or Q defect and need not necessarily mean the entire radiograph. A lung "zone" is one-third of the lung divided cranio-caudally. (Modified from Sostman HD, Rapoport S, Gottschalk A, et al. Imaging of pulmonary embolism. *Invest Radiol* 1986; 21:443-454. Reproduced by permission.)

3. The perfusion scan may be utilized by the angiographer to locate the lung region to study first, thus potentially decreasing the risk associated with the procedure by decreasing the amount of contrast utilized, decreasing the pressure and duration of the injection, and shortening the examination time.

Pulmonary Angiography

At present, pulmonary angiography is the "gold standard" diagnostic procedure for suspected PE. It is a safe procedure, with a mortality rate of 0.2%. Patients at relatively high risk for a fatal complication are those with right-ventricular end-diastolic pressures greater than 20 mm Hg. The nonfatal complication rate is approximately 3.5% to 5.5%.

Pulmonary angiography is usually performed after introduction of a pigtail catheter into the left or right pulmonary artery from a femoral vein. As the catheter is advanced toward the heart, repeated injections of contrast material should be made under fluoroscopic guidance to exclude thrombus in the iliac veins and IVC. If necessary, subselective injections of contrast material into lobar branches of the pulmonary arteries may be performed.

The only definitive angiographic signs of acute PE are the visualization of an embolus surrounded by contrast material within the vessel lumen, and the delineation of the trailing edge of an embolus obstructing a vessel. An abrupt cut-off of a vessel is not specific for PE, and this sign alone should not be used to diagnose PE. In addition, resolution of PE may result in permanent changes such as irregular vessel attenuation and webs within the lumen, hindering the distinction between an acute and previous, remote episode(s) of PE.

In general, angiography should be performed as soon after the diagnosis is suspected as practicable; this will decrease the possibility of complete lysis of emboli and a resultant false negative examination. However, there is no documented evidence that complete lysis will occur in 24 hours or less, so angiography may be safely deferred for several hours while the patient is stabilized and heparin therapy begun.

A Strategy for the Diagnosis of Pulmonary Embolism

When acute PE is initially suspected on the basis of clinical signs and symptoms, three diagnostic tests should be obtained: a chest radiograph; arterial blood gas analysis; and an electrocardiogram. If the results of these tests reveal a definite alternative cause for the patient's symptoms, such as a pneumothorax, myocardial infarction with cardiogenic pulmonary edema, or pneumonia, no further testing for PE is necessary. If PE is still a diagnostic consideration, a V/Q scan should be requested. At this point in the diagnostic process, a probabilistic estimate of the likelihood of PE should be made. For example, the absence of predisposing risk factors for PE coupled with an arterial oxygen pressure greater than 90 mm Hg in a patient with features otherwise suggestive of PE represents a very low likelihood of PE.

If the perfusion scan is normal, acute PE is excluded. If a high probability scan pattern is present in association with a high pretest estimate of the likelihood of PE, anticoagulation may be instituted. Pulmonary angiography should still be performed whenever one or more of the following issues pertain:

1. The patient is at high risk for hemorrhagic complications of conventional anticoagulant therapy (e.g., hemorrhagic diathesis; recent hemorrhagic cerebral infarction; bleeding peptic ulcer).

2. Localized or systemic fibrinolytic therapy is to be instituted.

3. Surgical ligation of the IVC or filter placement is to be performed. This applies particularly to patients with absolute or relative contraindications to anticoagulant therapy as described earlier.

If a low probability scan pattern is found in association with a low pretest estimate, pulmonary angiography and anticoagulation may be foregone.

If an intermediate probability or indeterminate scan pattern is found, pulmonary angiography should be performed unless an alternative cause for the patient's symptoms becomes apparent. An indeterminate scan is frequently found in patients with extensive emphysema, in whom greater than 50% of the lung fields show gas-trapping on the ventilation scan.

If the result of the V/Q scan and the pretest estimate of the likelihood of PE are discordant (e.g., a low probability scan pattern with a high pretest index of suspicion), pulmonary angiography should be performed.

This diagnostic strategy cannot be applied in isolation by the radiologist interpreting the imaging studies. Close communication with the physician responsible for the patient's management is essential.

CHRONIC (PROXIMAL) PULMONARY THROMBOEMBOLISM

Patients with this disorder may present initially with signs and symptoms of pulmonary hypertension, as described in chapter 4. In some patients, this may be the result of unresolved, proximal PE, with large clots present in the central pulmonary arteries. In other patients, in situ thrombosis may be responsible. Selected patients in this group may be candidates for surgical thromboembolectomy. If this diagnosis is considered, a V/Q scan should initially be obtained. If unmatched segmental/subsegmental defects are found, pulmonary angiography should be performed. The presence of central pulmonary artery thrombi may also be evaluated with dynamic, contrast material–enhanced computed tomography or magnetic resonance imaging.

Pulmonary Tumor Embolism

Embolism of tumor cells to the pulmonary microvascular bed may result in sufficient vascular occlusion to result in symptomatic pulmonary hypertension. Patients with extrapulmonary adenocarcinoma involving the breast, stomach, pancreas, kidney, and choriocarcinoma are typically affected. Rarely, tumor embolism may be the presenting manifestation of malignancy, with the site of origin remaining undetermined.

Patients typically present with progressively increasing dyspnea. Diagnostic tests reveal hypoxemia or a widened alveolar-to-arterial oxygen gradient, and clinical signs of pulmonary hypertension. As the differential diagnosis invariably includes bland pulmonary embolism, chest radiographs and a ventilation/perfusion scan are frequently obtained.

Radiography

In the majority of cases, the chest radiograph is normal. In a small number of patients, there are signs of so-called lymphangitic metastases to the lung: septal lines; small irregular shadows; small nodular shadows; peribronchial cuffs. Enlargement of the heart and central pulmonary arteries is infrequent.

A perfusion scan typically reveals inhomogeneous perfusion with small, nonsegmental defects. When numerous, these defects may appear to outline the margins of the bronchopulmonary segments. Segmental and true subsegmental defects are not a feature, and the ventilation scan is normal.

The combination of a normal chest radiograph and this V/Q scan pattern is very suggestive of tumor embolism in the appropriate setting. If histologic confirmation is required, this may be obtained by transbronchial or open lung biopsy. A recently described technique involves cytologic evaluation of blood drawn from a pulmonary artery occlusion catheter in the wedged position.

Pulmonary Fat Embolism

Pulmonary fat embolism is usually a sequel of long-bone fractures, with marrow fat gaining access to torn vessels at the fracture site. Fat emboli lodge in pulmonary microvessels, with resulting endothelial damage as toxic free fatty acids are produced through the action of pulmonary lipases on the fat globules. In severe cases, fat emboli pass into the systemic circulation to lodge in the cerebral, renal, and skin microvasculature. Patients may subsequently develop neurologic dysfunction, with confusion and a depressed level of consciousness, and skin petechiae.

Pulmonary fat embolism frequently becomes apparent after a latent period of 24 to 72 hours after the time of fracture. Increasing dyspnea and hypoxemia are the usual findings. The underlying pathologic abnormality is increased permeability pulmonary edema in association with diffuse alveolar damage. No specific treatment is available, and spontaneous resolution occurs in the vast majority of patients.

Radiography

The initial chest radiograph obtained may be normal despite clinical signs of respiratory distress and progressive hypoxemia. Thereafter, progressive, bilateral consolidation occurs. Diffuse, bilateral consolidation is the radiographic manifestation of increased-permeability pulmonary edema. Air bronchograms may be present, but septal lines are absent, and heart size is normal. Lung volumes decrease as lung edema increases, but are frequently modified by the application of positive pressure ventilation. If prolonged ventilatory support with high mean airway pressures becomes necessary, the radiograph should be evaluated for signs of barotrauma: pneumothorax, pneumomediastinum, and interstitial emphysema.

Pulmonary Septic Embolism

Septic embolism occurs in association with episodes of bacteremia or septicemia. Bacterial endocarditis affecting the tricuspid valve is the most common source of septic emboli, but emboli may arise from other sites of infection such as skin or subcutaneous tissue abscesses. Persons at highest risk are intravenous drug abusers and those with acquired abnormalities of the cardiac valves such as rheumatic tricuspid stenosis.

Septic emboli result in localized foci of parenchymal infection, predominantly in the lower lungs. If untreated, increasing areas of the lung become involved as "showers" of emboli lodge sequentially in multiple segments of the pulmonary vascular bed. Secondary involvement of the pleural space may occur with empyema formation.

Radiography

The radiographic appearance is one of multiple nodular opacities in both lungs. The nodules are usually not larger than 1 to 2 cm, and cavitation is a very common finding. If the patient is not adequately treated, localized areas of consolidation may develop. The appearance of pleural fluid may indicate development of an empyema. If endocarditis with valvular damage is the underlying cause, radiographic signs of congestive heart failure may be present.

SELECTED REFERENCES

Alderson PO, Martin EC: Pulmonary embolism: Diagnosis with multiple imaging modalities. *Radiology* 1987; 164:297.

Batra P: The fat embolism syndrome. *J Thorac Imag* 1987; 2(3):12.

Chan CK, Hutcheon MA, Hyland RH, et al: Pulmonary tumor embolism: A critical review of clinical, imaging and hemodynamic features. *J Thorac Imag* 1987; 2(4):4.

Fisher MR, Higgins CB: Central thrombi in pulmonary artery hypertension detected by MR imaging. *Radiology* 1986; 158:223.

Greenspan RH, Ravin CE, Polansky SM, et al: Accuracy of chest radiograph in diagnosis of pulmonary embolism *Invest Radiol* 1982; 17:539.

Kereiakes DJ, Herfkens RJ, Brundage BH, et al: Computerized tomography in chronic thromboembolic pulmonary hypertension *Am Heart J* 1983; 106:1432.

Sostman HD, Rapoport S, Gottschalk A, et al: Imaging of pulmonary embolism. *Invest Radiol* 1986; 21:443.

Woodruff WW, Hoeck BE, Chitwood WR, et al: Radiographic findings in pulmonary hypertension from unresolved emboli. *AJR* 1985; 144:681.

6

The Trachea

Howard Mann, M.D.

KEY CONCEPTS

1. Common causes of diffuse tracheal narrowing are infectious and noninfectious granulomatous diseases.
2. Tracheal amyloid should be suspected when calcified submucosal nodules are identified.
3. There is an association between a saber-sheath trachea (tracheal index less than 0.5) and chronic obstructive airways disease.
4. Suspected tracheomalacia should be evaluated fluoroscopically.

TRACHEAL DIMENSIONS

The tracheal rings are generally semicircular in construction, being C- or U-shaped, and determine the cross-sectional appearance of the trachea. Separate coronal and sagittal diameters may be defined. The tracheal index is a ratio of the coronal and sagittal diameters. Normally, this ratio is close to 1:1. A summary of the most common benign causes of abnormal widening and narrowing is presented in Table 6-1.

DIFFUSE TRACHEAL NARROWING

Fungal Infections

In the category of fungal infections, histoplasmosis, coccidioidomycosis, candidiasis, and phycomycosis

TABLE 6–1.
Causes of Diffuse Tracheal Narrowing and Widening

Diffuse Tracheal Narrowing	Diffuse Tracheal Widening
Fungal infections	Mounier-Kühn syndrome
Tuberculosis	Ehlers-Danlos syndrome
Wegener's granulomatosis	Cutis laxa
Relapsing polychondritis	Ataxia telangiectasia
Sarcoidosis	Relapsing polychondritis (rare)
Amyloidosis	
Tracheopathia osteochondroplastica	
Saber-sheath trachea	
Idiopathic mediastinal fibrosis	

should be considered. Overall, an intrinsic stenosing process causing luminal narrowing is a rare feature of fungal infections involving the respiratory tract. As described in the chapter on pulmonary infections, granulomatous fibrosing mediastinitis resulting from histoplasmosis may cause tracheal narrowing, along with compression/stenosis of other mediastinal vascular structures.

Tuberculosis

Trachea narrowing is much less common than stricture formation involving the proximal bronchi. More focal stenosis may result from secondary involvement by adjacent infected lymph nodes.

Wegener's Granulomatosis

Upper respiratory tract involvement is an almost invariable feature of this disease. Paranasal sinus disease is much more common, but occasional isolated cases of tracheal involvement have been reported. The stenosis usually begins in the subglottic space.

Relapsing Polychondritis

This disease of unknown cause is typically characterized by episodic, recurrent bouts of inflammation involving cartilaginous structures in many sites. It affects both sexes and usually manifests in the 3rd or 4th decade of life. A particularly common site of symptomatic involvement is the cartilage of the external ear (pinna); other sites include the nasal, laryngeal, tracheal, and articular cartilages. Pathologically, there is loss of basophilic staining and metachromasia of the cartilage matrix, which appears to be the result of loss of acid mucopolysaccharides. Recurrent bouts of inflammation result in progressive scarring, but the time course of the disease is highly variable. The importance of upper respiratory tract disease is that progressive narrowing of the airway may cause severe disability and death. Uncommonly, destruction of tracheal cartilages results in functional tracheomalacia, with collapse on expiration and variable widening on inspiration.

Sarcoidosis

Tracheal involvement is much less common than laryngeal sarcoidosis. Distal extension from the subglottic space may occur.

Amyloidosis

Tracheobronchial amyloidosis may present with localized, nodular masses of tissue within the lumen of the airway or as diffuse narrowing. In the latter instance, submucosal deposits of amyloid protein typically produce focal elevations of the mucosal surface, easily visible on bronchoscopy. This permits diagnosis by bronchoscopically directed biopsy. Focal calcification within amyloid protein may occur.

Tracheopathia Osteochondroplastica

This rare disorder is characterized by the presence of localized submucosal foci of osteocartilagenous tissue. The posterior membranous trachea is rarely involved. The submucosal nodules protrude into and deform the lumen. In this respect, the condition closely resembles amyloidosis. Calcification of cartilaginous and osseous matrix is common, and thus permits the diagnosis on conventional or computed tomography. This is a disorder of the elderly, and may be an incidental finding on chest radiographs.

Saber-Sheath Trachea

This term describes the finding of a decreased coronal diameter of the trachea, with a tracheal index less than 0.5. While this may occasionally be an incidental finding in elderly men, it has an important association with chronic obstructive airways disease. Typically, the diameter of the trachea abruptly decreases as it passes through the thoracic inlet, and becomes exposed to intrathoracic pressure; thus the proximal site of narrowing is usually opposite the first costomanubrial junction on the frontal radiograph.

Idiopathic Mediastinal Fibrosis

This form of fibrosis may also result in compression/narrowing of other mediastinal structures, particularly the superior and inferior vena cavae. Tracheal narrowing rarely occurs alone. In this respect, it is similar to granulomatous fibrosing mediastinitis due to histoplasmosis. Importantly, there is an association with retroperitoneal fibrosis, which may occlude the ureters, and with methysergide therapy.

DIFFUSE TRACHEAL WIDENING

Mounier-Kühn Syndrome (Tracheobronchomegaly)

This disorder may be suspected when the coronal diameter of the trachea is ≥3 cm, and that of the mainstem bronchi is ≥2.5 cm. It is a disorder of the elderly and is associated with chronic lower respiratory tract infections, possibly due to diminished clearance of secretions by the mucociliary escalator in the presence of abnormal expiratory collapse of the central airways. The latter may be observed during fluoroscopic examination. On the lateral radiograph, prominent invagination of the tracheal wall between the cartilaginous rings may sometimes be observed. The cause of this disorder is unknown, but may represent a congenital defect in the elastic and muscular fibers of the tracheal wall.

Tracheal Dilatation in Disorders of Connective Tissue

Not surprisingly, tracheomegaly has been reported in association with Ehlers-Danlos syndrome and aquired cutis laxa. Thus, there may be a similarity in terms of pathogenesis with the Mounier-Kühn syndrome described earlier.

RADIOGRAPHIC ASSESSMENT OF TRACHEAL MORPHOLOGY

Assessment may be accomplished with radiographs

collimated to the area of interest, and with conventional and computed (CT) tomography. CT scanning is an excellent means of evaluating tracheal disease, particularly because it allows assessment of the adjacent extratracheal mediastinal tissues. Conventional linear tomography is very useful in evaluating the extent of narrowing when a diffuse process is present, and is probably superior to CT scanning in this regard.

FLUOROSCOPIC ASSESSMENT OF TRACHEAL DYNAMICS

Fluoroscopy may provide unique and diagnostic information when abnormal collapsibility of the trachea is present; for example, in acquired tracheomalacia resulting from tracheal wall damage as a result of endotracheal intubation. A videotape recording of the examination may be made for later analysis and documentation. This means of evaluation may complement bronchoscopic examination of the trachea.

SELECTED REFERENCES

Lechner GL, Jantsch HS, Greene RG: Radiology of the trachea, in Taveras JM, Ferrucci, JT (eds): *Radiology, Diagnosis-Imaging-Intervention*. Philadelphia, JB Lippincott Co, 1986, vol 1.

Choplin RH, Wehunt WD, Theros EG: Diffuse lesions of the trachea. *Semin Roentgenol* 1983; 18(1):38.

Greene RE: Saber-sheath trachea: Relation to chronic obstructive pulmonary disease. *AJR* 1978; 130:441.

Kilman WJ: Narrowing of the airway in relapsing polychrondritis. *Radiology* 1978; 126:373.

Young RH, Sandstrom RE, Mark GJ: Tracheopathia osteoplastica: Clinical, radiologic, and pathologic correlations. *J Thorac Cardiovasc Surg* 1980; 70:537.

7

Chronic Bronchial Disease

Howard Mann, M.D.

KEY CONCEPTS

1. The term "chronic obstructive airways disease" refers to the presence of chronic expiratory airflow limitation. It is not a radiographic diagnosis.
2. Chronic bronchitis is associated with the development of pulmonary hypertension, which may be evident on a chest radiograph.
3. Cystic bronchiectasis produces cystic spaces containing fluid (demilunes) on the chest radiograph.
4. Mucus plugs in chronic asthma may produce rounded, oval, and tubular shadows on the chest radiograph.
5. Bronchiectasis is usually most severe in the lower lungs except in cystic fibrosis, when upper lobe involvement is predominant.
6. Bronchiolitis obliterans, organizing pneumonia may produce localized areas of consolidation, typically in a "ground-glass" pattern.

DEFINITIONS AND PATHOPHYSIOLOGY

The clinical manifestations of diseases in this category reflect the presence of two primary pathophysiologic abnormalities: expiratory airflow limitation and excessive mucus production. The relative importance of these two features will vary both between diseases and individual patients.

The term "chronic obstructive airways disease" encompasses three disorders characterized by expiratory airflow limitation: emphysema; chronic bronchitis; and peripheral airways disease. Asthma is excluded from this definition, as expiratory airflow in this condition is reversible. Bronchiolitis obliterans affects primarily terminal and respiratory bronchioles, but involvement of alveolar ducts and alveoli may be present in bronchiolitis obliterans, organizing pneumonia. Bronchiectasis and cystic fibrosis are characterized by excessive mucus production, repeated infections and bronchial dilatation.

CHRONIC BRONCHITIS

Chronic bronchitis has been defined strictly in clinical terms as a condition associated with mucus hypersecretion from the bronchial glands, and a consequent chronic, productive cough occurring for at least 3 months of the year for at least 2 successive years.

Pathologically, there is hyperplasia of bronchial mucous glands, with an increased ratio reflecting the width of the mucous glands relative to the width of the bronchial wall—the Reid Index. In addition, there is often more distal extension of goblet cells along the bronchial tree than usual.

Chronic hypoxia is typically associated with hypercarbia and cyanosis ("blue bloater"). Pulmonary hypertension and cor pulmonale are the usual causes of death.

Radiography

Unlike the situation with pulmonary emphysema, there is a lack of radiologic-pathologic correlative studies in this disorder. Hence, the traditional concept of increased "bronchovascular markings" as diagnostic of this condition remains controversial. This concept emphasizes the presumed underlying pathologic condition of bronchial dilatation with bronchial wall thickening, and dilated pulmonary arteries due to arterial hypertension. Of course, signs of coexistent emphysema may be present, as well as central pulmonary artery dilatation and enlargement of the right side of the heart. In the era of bronchography, this disorder was diagnosed by opacifying the dilated necks of enlarged mucous glands in the walls of the larger bronchi.

The diagnosis of chronic bronchitis should be suspected whenever a chest radiograph reveals evidence of pulmonary arterial hypertension without hyperinflated lungs. Clinical information should be obtained, particularly with respect to chronic hypoxia, excessive mucus production, and repeated pulmonary infections. The differential diagnosis includes the alveolar hypoventilation/sleep apnea syndromes.

ASTHMA

In asthma there is evidence of bronchial muscle hyperreactivity with reversible episodes of bronchial constriction. The onset of wheezing reflects the occurrence of an allergic, type I immune response to a specific allergen or allergens.

In chronic asthma, there may be pathologic evidence of smooth muscle hypertrophy, bronchial wall thickening, and bronchial dilatation in association with occlusive mucus plugs.

Radiography

Findings on chest radiography may be divided into two categories: those reflecting the underlying primary pathologic process, and those reflecting the potential complications of that process:

Category 1

1. Bronchial dilatation. This is usually evident when a bronchial segment is filled with mucus, and is evident as a focal tubular opacity which may branch in a "Y" configuration. If there is cystic bronchiectasis, an oval or rounded opacity will be seen.

2. Bronchial wall thickening. This is classically described in the presence of two thin, parallel lines seen in the distribution of central, segmental bronchi. These "tram tracks" represent air in the bronchial lumen between thickened bronchial walls. This may also be seen as small circular shadows, "bronchial cuffing," when the bronchi are viewed en face.

Category 2

1. Atelectasis. Variable areas of atelectasis may occur proximal to bronchial obstruction caused by mucus plugs. Typically, segmental or lobar atelectasis occurs, and this may rapidly resolve when these mucus plugs are expectorated.
2. Consolidation. This is due to complicating pneumonia and may be associated with the obstructive volume loss.
3. Pneumomediastinum and pneumothorax. These may occur during an acute episode of bronchospasm with attendent air-trapping and lung overinflation. Air dissects from the alveoli into the interstitial space of the alveolar septa, and thence proximally along the bronchovascular sheaths into the mediastinum. Air may dissect toward the pleural surface to form blebs of interstitial emphysema within the layers of the visceral pleura. Subsequent rupture into the pleural space may occur, giving rise to a pneumothorax.
4. Pulmonary arterial hypertension. This may occur in severe, chronic asthma and manifest with dilated central pulmonary arteries.

ALLERGIC BRONCHOPULMONARY ASPERGILLOSIS

This particular entity may be seen in otherwise normal individuals, but is much more prevalent in those with chronic asthma. This disorder was described in the section on pulmonary infections, and is summarized in Table 7–1.

TABLE 7-1.
Criteria for the Diagnosis of Allergic Bronchopulmonary Aspergillosis

Clinical/Serologic	Radiographic
Asthma	Bronchial dilatation
Peripheral eosinophilia	Bronchial mucus plugs
Elevated serum IgE	Areas of atelectasis
Precipitating serum Abs* to aspergillus	Cavitation/mycetoma formation (uncommon)
Immediate skin reaction to aspergillus	
Aspergillus hyphae in mucus plugs	

*Abs = IgG antibodies.

It is important to make the diagnosis of this disorder, as steroid therapy will prevent recurrent acute episodes and the complications of pulmonary fibrosis and bronchiectasis. If there is any doubt about the presence of bronchial dilatation/mucus plugging, conventional linear or computed (CT) tomography may be performed, which will demonstrate these findings to better advantage.

BRONCHIECTASIS

Bronchiectasis shares many features with chronic bronchitis and asthma, but its most distinguishing characteristic is its tendency to be localized to a lobe or lung region. Thus, surgical resection of an involved area of lung may be curative.

When this diagnosis is made for the first time, the cause is often not apparent. It is presumed that most cases follow an episode/s of infection in early life with associated structural damage to the bronchial wall.

As with emphysema, the generally accepted classification is based on morphologic findings evident on bronchography, which rarely needs to be performed today in the era of bronchoscopy and CT scanning.

Reid's classification involves three groups:

1. Cylindric bronchiectasis. Bronchi are only mildly dilated and retain their tubular shape. The pattern of dichotomous branching appears normal
2. Varicose bronchiectasis. Greater, generalized dilatation is present, and localized, bulbous areas of dilatation are evident. The number of patent subdivisions is reduced.
3. Cystic bronchiectasis. In this form, cystic, rounded spaces are present. The number of subdivisions does not usually exceed five.

Patients with bronchiectasis usually present with a history of recurrent bouts of pneumonia with or without associated hemoptysis. In severe cases, patients expectorate large amounts of foul-smelling, purulent sputum.

Radiography

Mild forms of cylindric and varicose bronchiectasis will be associated with a normal radiograph. In the appropriate clinical setting, the diagnosis may be suggested when thickened bronchial walls are seen in the absence of other causes for this finding such as chronic bronchitis, asthma, cystic fibrosis, and allergic bronchopulmonary aspergillosis. Cystic bronchiectasis is more easily diagnosed when larger cystic spaces are seen, particularly in association with fluid levels within the dilated bronchi, so-called demilunes.

When it is important to establish the extent and distribution of disease, CT scanning is the initial examination of choice: dilated bronchi are visible as ring shadows adjacent to corresponding branches of the pulmonary arterial tree; a signet-ring appearance is characteristic. As the predictive values of CT are relatively low in the presence of mild cylindric/varicose bronchiectasis, bronchography may still be indicated when the clinical suspicion of disease is high. Finally, whenever a cystic pattern is present on chest radiographs, care should be taken not to mistake cystic bronchiectasis for the cystic spaces and/or honeycombing of interstitial fibrosis. The latter is never associated with fluid levels, and bronchiectasis generally involves the lower lobes.

PRIMARY CILIARY DYSKINESIA

Patients with primary ciliary dyskinesia have chronic sinusitis, otitis, and bronchitis/bronchiectasis. Affected males are typically infertile due to defective sperm motility. The underlying cause is a genetic defect resulting in abnormal movement of cilia and inadequate clearance of secretions from mucosal surfaces. Kartagener's syndrome refers to the presence of bronchiectasis with dextrocardia and situs inversus, although not all affected persons have the complete triad. Radiographically, this disorder presents as a relatively mild form of cystic fibrosis.

CYSTIC FIBROSIS

This disorder is characterized by an autosomal recessive mode of inheritance, abnormally high levels of sodium and chloride in sweat, and chronic pancreatic and pulmonary disease. The basic defect is in the secretory process, with resultant pancreatic exocrine insufficiency and chronic airflow obstruction.

Chronic pulmonary disease presents usually as a chronic cough, with or without wheezing. Recurrent lower respiratory infection is common, and organisms such as mucoid *Pseudomonas* and *Staphylococcus aureus* chronically colonize the lower respiratory tract. Chronic airway obstruction by viscid secretions leads to hyperinflation, bronchiectasis, areas of atelectasis, recurrent pneumonia, and finally pulmonary vascular hypertension/cor pulmonale. Hemoptysis is a common complication and may be life threatening. Bleeding is thought to originate from dilated bronchial-pulmonary vascular anastomoses about foci of chronic infection. Pneumothorax is another fairly common occurrence, reflecting a severe bout of air-trapping.

Radiography

The spectrum of findings is very similar to that of chronic bronchitis and asthma. A very characteristic finding is the predominant involvement of the upper lobes, particularly early in the course of the disease. Another important presentation involves patients with a very mild form of cystic fibrosis who present for the first time as young adults: radiographic findings may consist only of bronchial wall thickening and linear/irregular nonvascular shadows in the upper lobes, along with unexplained chronic, mild hyperinflation.

A high index of suspicion is necessary to make the diagnosis. The typical radiographic findings and corresponding structural abnormalities are summarized in Table 7–2.

BRONCHIOLITIS OBLITERANS

This is a disorder that affects the distal airways and bronchioles, and produces clinically significant airflow obstruction. In some cases, there is also a decrease in diffusing capacity, particularly when there is a prominent interstitial fibrotic component. Most patients present with an insidious onset of cough and dyspnea.

On pathologic examination, there is often evidence of granulation tissue plugs within the lumina of respiratory bronchioles, with extension into alveolar ducts and alveoli. Hence the term "bronchiolitis obliterans, organizing pneumonia" is commonly employed, clearly separating this entity from usual interstitial pneumonia.

The classification reflects the known etiologies, including an idiopathic variety:

1. Toxic fume exposure. Chlorine and phosgene, for example, are known causes (pure bronchiolitis obliterans).
2. Postinfectious. Adenoviral and mycoplasma infections have been implicated.
3. Connective tissue disease. Rheumatoid arthritis is an important association.
4. Localized. Usually an incidental finding in association with other lesions such as carcinoma (pure bronchiolitis obliterans).
5. Idiopathic.

It is important to distinguish this entity from usual interstitial pneumonitis, as steroid therapy may result in marked improvement, particularly in the idiopathic variety.

TABLE 7-2.
Radiographic Diagnosis of Cystic Fibrosis*

Radiographic Findings	Structural Abnormality
Hyperinflation	Bronchial obstruction by viscid mucus
Ring shadows	Bronchiectasis/bronchial wall thickening
Tram-tracks	Bronchial wall thickening
Peripheral small nodular shadows	Small bronchi distended with mucus
Areas of atelectasis	Bronchial luminal occlusion by mucus
Cystic spaces	Cystic bronchiectasis/cavitation due to recurrent infection and abscess formation
Hilar enlargement	Pulmonary artery and/or lymph node enlargment

*Modified from Pagtakhan RD, Reed MH, Chernick V: Cystic fibrosis in the adolescent and adult. *J Thorac Imaging* 1986; 4:41-48. Reproduced by permission of Aspen Publishers, Inc.

Radiography

In some cases the radiograph may be normal, particularly when a relatively pure form of bronchiolitis is present. When associated with a connective tissue disease, it may be an unsuspected finding on a histologic specimen, while the radiograph shows the typical findings expected with that disorder. In the idiopathic variety, the radiograph often shows a typical "ground-glass" opacity in both lungs: the opacity is usually poorly marginated and does not conform to segmental or lobar boundaries. Uncommonly, a mixture of linear and irregular opacities may be seen.

When an obliterative bronchiolitis follows a childhood infection, a distinct constellation of abnormalities may result, giving rise to a unilateral hyperlucent lung on radiography—the Swyer-James or Macleod's syndrome. This may be distinguished from other causes of this radiographic phenomenon, such as the hypogenetic lung syndrome, by obtaining a radiograph in expiration, which will reveal air-trapping on the affected side. Other findings on chest radiographs include cystic spaces due to emphysematous bullae forming proximal to narrowed bronchioles. Ventilation/perfusion scintigraphy will reveal absent ventilation and perfusion to the affected lung.

SELECTED REFERENCES

Blair DN, Coppage L, Shaw C: Medical imaging in asthma. *J Thorac Imag* 1986; 1(2): 23.

Chandler PW, Shin MS, Friedman SE, et al: Radiographic manifestations of bronchiolitis obliterans with organizing pneumonia. *AJR* 1986; 147:899.

Cooke JC, Currie DC, Morgan AD, et al: Role of computed tomography in diagnosis of bronchiectasis. *Thorax* 1987; 42:272.

Epler GR, Colby TV, McCloud TC, et al: Bronchiolitis obliterans organizing pneumonia. *N Engl J Med* 1985; 312:152.

Mintzer RA, Rogers LF, Kruglick GD, et al: The spectrum of radiologic findings in allergic bronchopulmonary aspergillosis. *Radiology* 1978; 127:301.

Nadel HR, Stringer DA, Levinson H, et al: The immotile cilia syndrome: Radiological manifestations *Radiology* 1985; 154:651.

Pagtakhan RD, Reed MH, Chernick V: Cystic fibrosis in the adolescent and adult. *J Thorac Imag* 1986; 1(4):41.

Reid LM: Reduction in bronchial subdivisions in bronchiectasis. *Thorax* 1950; 5:233.

8

Emphysema

Howard Mann, M.D.

KEY CONCEPTS

1. The definition of emphysema reflects abnormal parenchymal morphology.
2. A chest radiograph may be used to diagnose or exclude emphysema, not chronic obstructive pulmonary disease.
3. The cardinal signs of emphysema are hyperinflation and localized radiolucent areas associated with vascular attenuation/obliteration.
4. Severe basal emphysema is typically found in α-1-antitrypsin deficiency.
5. In the presence of emphysema, pulmonary edema will be localized to areas of normally perfused lung.
6. Consolidation involving emphysematous areas of lung will be very inhomogeneous on chest radiography.

DEFINITION

Emphysema is a condition characterized by an increase beyond the normal size of air spaces distal to the terminal bronchiole, without significant fibrosis. As this is primarily a pathologic description, emphysema is not a single disease, but a manifestation of many etiologies. The pathogenesis most well appreciated, at least as it relates to panacinar emphysema, involves an imbalance between proteases and protease-inhibitors in the lung. The protease primarily implicated is neutrophil elastase, which degrades lung elastin, leading to alveolar wall destruction. Smoking is a well-known cause of emphysema, but the precise mechanism or mechanisms by which it promotes emphysema is not well understood.

MORPHOLOGIC CATEGORIES

Four major morphologic categories of emphysema may be considered: (1) centrilobular emphysema; (2) panacinar emphysema; (3) paraseptal emphysema; and (4) irregular emphysema. This anatomic classification is useful as a means of pathologic description, but the clinical/functional effects will depend on the extent and distribution of the emphysematous change in the lung and on the presence of coexistent conditions such as chronic bronchitis and asthma.

Centrilobular (Centriacinar) Emphysema

This form initially involves the alveoli that arise directly from the respiratory bronchiole, and is thus located in the center of the pulmonary acinus—that portion of lung air space distal to a terminal bronchiole. This form of emphysema is distributed in regions of maximum gravitational stress and sharp radii of curvature, particularly in the apical portions of the upper lobes. Centrilobar emphysema is by far the most common of the four pathologic types, and is not uncommonly seen in mild form in the lung apices of asymptomatic persons.

Panacinar Emphysema

This form involves the entire acinus and is frequently a cause of clinical disability. It may involve predominantly the lower lungs in α_1-antitrypsin deficiency, be regionally asymmetric, or be bilateral and diffuse. Panacinar emphysema is responsible for a mild form of "senile" emphysema that may be seen in the aged. This form of emphysema may be recognized readily on chest radiograph, as will be described later.

Paraseptal Emphysema

As its name implies, paraseptal emphysema represents dilatation of air spaces in the peripheral portions of the secondary pulmonary lobule, adjacent to the interlobular septa and connective tissue sheaths of the bronchovascular bundles. It is believed that a severe form of this emphysema is responsible for the condition of "vanishing lung disease," in which very large emphysematous spaces are associated with severe compression of adjacent, normal lung. Certain patients in this group may be candidates for surgical bullectomy. In general, however, it is usually recognized only on pathologic examination or computed tomographic scanning.

Irregular Emphysema

This is a localized form of paracicatricial (scar) emphysema surrounding a focal fibrotic process or tumor. A prime example is the focal emphysema surrounding the conglomerate masses (progressive massive fibrosis) of complicated silicosis.

RADIOGRAPHY

The radiographic detection of emphysema depends on the recognition of morphologic/structural abnormalities characteristic of this disease. Chronic obstructive pulmonary disease (COPD) is a clinical diagnosis based primarily on the presence of expiratory airflow limitation, determined on the basis of physical and spirometric examination. Included in this definition are emphysema, chronic bronchitis and peripheral airways disease (primarily bronchiolitis obliterans). On the basis of a chest radiograph, a radiologist may be able to diagnose or exclude emphysema, but not COPD.

The radiographic diagnosis of emphysema relates to the presence of two cardinal morphologic abnormalities that are manifest on a chest radiograph:

1. Increased total lung capacity—lung hyperinflation;

2. Formation of bullae—irregular radiolucency with vascular attenuation.

Lung Hyperinflation

Hyperinflation is the primary sign of emphysema, and may be diagnosed when the following are present: flattened hemidiaphragms; increased retrosternal airspace; and increased retrocardiac airspace. Flattened hemidiaphragms will manifest on the lateral projection as a sternodiaphragmatic angle of greater than 90 degrees. On the frontal projection, the costal slips of the hemidiaphragms may be visible. The heart may appear small relative to the size of the thorax. The patient's body habitus should be taken into account when assessing lung volumes—the apparently "large" lungs of a tall, thin person should not be mistaken for pathologic hyperinflation.

Radiolucent Areas With Vascular Attenuation

Bullae may be visible as rounded, cystic spaces devoid of normal vascular shadows. The margins of bullae may be seen as extremely thin, curvilinear opacities. An indirect sign of underlying bullae formation is irregular, peripheral attenuation of pulmonary vessels. The tubular shadows of vessels may end abruptly, and there is a loss of normal dichotomous branching.

The positive and negative predictive values of these radiographic features is high when the prevalence of emphysema in the population studied is above 5%, a common situation. Thus, chest radiography is a useful means of diagnosing or excluding the presence of morphologic emphysema in the patient known to have COPD.

PULMONARY HYPERTENSION IN EMPHYSEMA

Pulmonary hypertension may be diagnosed when there is dilatation of the central main, left, and right pulmonary arteries. The caliber of pulmonary vessels in the upper lobes will increase as intraluminal pressure increases, and this will be most evident with the patient in the erect position as the caliber of upper lobe arteries approaches that of lower lobe vessels. Pulmonary hypertension will also cause "pruning" of the arterial tree, contributing to the peripheral attenuation of pulmonary vessels described earlier.

Cor pulmonale will be associated with progressive hypertrophy and dilatation of the right chamber; this is best appreciated in comparison with previous radiographs.

PULMONARY EDEMA AND PNEUMONIA IN EMPHYSEMA

The presence of emphysema will alter the usual appearance of pneumonia and pulmonary edema. In the case of consolidation due to pneumonia, the involved area will manifest very inhomogeneous opacity as alveolar fluid surrounds variably-sized cystic areas; a "swiss-cheese" appearance may be evident. The appearance of pulmonary edema will be similar, but its distribution will be determined by the distribution of blood flow in both lungs. The result may be very asymmetric and localized areas of edema, with sparing of zones of emphysematous lung. Comparison with previous radiographs obtained during an episode of cardiac failure will be very helpful.

COMPUTED TOMOGRAPHY IN EMPHYSEMA

The role of CT in the evaluation of a patient with emphysema is limited: its one established role is in the work-up of a patient for surgical bullectomy, as mentioned previously. In this instance it has replaced angiography as a means of evaluating the areas of compressed lung for evidence of widespread bullous disease, which would be a contraindication to surgery.

SELECTED REFERENCES

Carr DH, Pride NB: Computed tomography in preoperative assessment of bullous emphysema. *Clin Radiol* 1984; 35:43.

Greene RE, Reid R: Pulmonary emphysema, bullae, blebs, and lung cysts, in Taveras JM, Ferrucci JT (eds): *Radiology, Diagnosis-Imaging-Intervention.* Philadelphia, JB Lippincott Co, 1986, vol 1.

Hublitz UF, Shapiro JH: Atypical pulmonary patterns of congestive failure in chronic lung disease. *Radiology* 1969; 93:995.

Morgan MDL, Denison DM, Strickland B: Value of computed tomography for selecting patients with bullous disease for surgery. *Thorax* 1986; 41:855.

Pratt PC: Role of conventional chest radiograph in diagnosis and exclusion of emphysema. *Am J Med* 1987; 82:998.

9

Occupational Lung Disease

Howard Mann, M.D.

KEY CONCEPTS

1. Calcified and noncalcified pleural plaques are markers of previous asbestos exposure, having occurred at least 15 to 20 years previously.
2. Other pleural manifestations of asbestos exposure include asbestos-related effusion, diffuse pleural thickening, rounded atelectasis, and malignant mesothelioma.
3. Interstitial fibrosis due to asbestos (asbestosis) takes the form of basal small, irregular shadows.
4. Simple silicosis and coal-worker's pneumoconiosis produce small, nodular shadows (usually 1.5 to 3 mm) in the upper lobes. Complicated disease produces large opacities (progressive massive fibrosis) with irregular emphysema.
5. Chronic berylliosis is a granulomatous disorder and is radiographically indistinguishable from sarcoidosis.
6. Hypersensitivity pneumonitis is diagnosed on the basis of typical signs and symptoms associated with an appropriate exposure history. A chest radiograph may be normal.

This section will focus on lung diseases associated with occupational exposure to specific organic and inorganic substances. Only the most prevalent and clinically important diseases will be covered under the following broad categories: (1) inorganic dust pneumoconioses, and (2) hypersensitivity pneumonitis.

INORGANIC DUST PNEUMOCONIOSIS

In North America, three distinct disorders account for the vast majority of fibrotic, disabling lung diseases resulting from exposure to inorganic particles or fibers in the workplace: asbestosis and asbestos-related pleural disease, silicosis, and coal-worker's pneumoconiosis. Exposure to nonfibrogenic substances such as iron, tin, barium, and antimony rarely lead to functional disability, even though nodular shadows may be seen diffusely throughout the lung on chest radiography. These nonfibrogenic disorders will not be discussed further.

Asbestosis

Asbestos is a generic term that applies to a number of different hydrous silicates. In the United States, 90% of the asbestos used is chrysotile (white asbestos), which consists of wavy, serpiginous fibers. The straight fibers (amphiboles) include crocidolite (blue asbestos), amosite, tremolite, and anthophyllite. Crocidolite fibers have the smallest diameters, facilitating penetration into the distal bronchial tree; crocidolite exposure is associated with the highest incidence of pleural and peritoneal mesotheliomas. Importantly, commercial talc contains significant quantities of anthophyllite and tremolite, accounting for the observed occurrence of pleural disease resulting from exposure to this fibrous silicate.

Epidemiology

The mining and milling of asbestos is not an important source of exposure to asbestos in North America today. Exposure occurs in industries that manufacture or use asbestos-containing products. Exposure still occurs in the construction industry. Even a relatively brief, but intense, exposure to asbestos may result in pleural disease after a latent period of 20 to 40 years. Thus, very close and detailed questioning of the patient may be necessary to uncover a source of exposure that may have been overlooked or forgotten. Contamination of a worker's clothes may result in significant exposure to his/her spouse and children in the home environment.

Pathogenesis

A linear dose-response exists between the cumulative amount of inhaled fibers and the development of asbestos-related disease, particularly interstitial fibrosis. However, many additional factors such as individual genetic susceptibility and immunologic responsiveness also play a role, as yet not clearly defined.

Inhaled asbestos fibers, 3 μm or less in diameter, penetrate as far as the respiratory bronchioles and alveoli. Fibers that reach the alveoli tend to remain there throughout the subject's life, and may become coated with a ferritin-like protein to form ferruginous bodies that may be seen on light microscopy. However, ferruginous bodies are not specific for asbestos fibers.

Asbestos fibers may cause both pleural and parenchymal abnormalities, and these will be discussed separately.

Asbestos-Related Pleural Disease

Several distinct abnormalities related to pleural space disease have been described: asbestos-related effusion; pleural plaques; diffuse pleural thickening; rounded atelectasis; and malignant mesothelioma.

Asbestos-Related Pleural Effusion

Recurrent, cytologically benign effusions may occur with or without symptoms. Symptoms include chest pain and dyspnea if the effusion is large. Aspirated fluid may be serosanguinous with pleural fluid eosinophilia. These effusions may occur long before the appearance of pleural plaques, and be the first indication of previous asbestos exposure. The effusions may resolve completely or leave a variable amount of pleural thickening, such as blunting of the costophrenic angles. Some authorities consider these effusions to be "premalignant," particularly if they are recurrent, and these patients should be observed closely because of the known risk of malignant mesothelioma formation.

Pleural Plaques

Calcified and noncalcified pleural plaques may be considered specific evidence of previous asbestos exposure, although exposure to other minerals such as zeolites is a recognized rare cause. Typically, there is a latent period of at least 15–20 years between the exposure (which may have occurred over a period of several months only) and the appearance of plaques on conventional radiography. These plaques do not cause symptoms. They are usually found along the midportion of the lateral chest wall and along the hemidiaphragmatic pleural surfaces. They are not generally seen in the apices or the costophrenic angles. Plaques may enlarge slowly, but it usually takes 3 to 5 years for a change in size to be apparent.

Pleural plaques are located on the parietal pleural surface. They consist of acellular collagenous tissue, and asbestos fibers are not seen on light microscopy. At autopsy, many more plaques are found than are apparent on conventional radiography.

Radiography.—Plaques appear as focal, circumscribed opacities that may or may not appear calcified. When seen in profile, they have a characteristic flat, linear configuration. When seen *en face*, they are irregular in shape, with ill-defined margins. In this configuration, they often appear inhomogeneous in density because of variable calcification within the plaque. When doubt exists concerning the presence of plaques, fluoroscopy with low (65) kV(p) spot radiographs in varying degrees of obliquity should be performed. If this technique does not resolve the question, computed tomography (CT) of the chest may be performed.

Several entities may simulate plaques or localized pleural thickening on conventional radiographs:

1. Healed rib fractures;
2. Focal accumulation of subcostal fat (usually symmetric, in obese patients);
3. Costal slips of the serratus anterior muscle; and
4. Soft-tissue companion shadows (internal intercostal muscle plus fat).

These may be differentiated by obtaining oblique views and/or by fluoroscopy. If necessary, CT scanning may be performed.

Diffuse Pleural Thickening

Diffuse pleural thickening involves the visceral pleura, particularly in association with diffuse interstitial fibrosis. This most likely represents the interstitial process extending to the subpleural space with secondary involvement of the pleura. Diffuse thickening extending upwards from a costophrenic angle may also represent a sequel of recurrent effusions described earlier. Thickening of the pleura in the interlobar fissures represents exclusive visceral pleural involvement, and may be seen in the apparent absence of interstitial fibrosis. Unilateral, diffuse pleural thickening, particularly with extensive calcification, is not a feature of asbestos-related disease; other causes such as empyema and trauma (hemothorax) should be considered.

Rounded Atelectasis or Atelectatic Pseudotumor

This localized parenchymal abnormality is frequently mistaken for primary bronchogenic carcinoma. It is thought to represent a sequel of chronic pleural effusion and pleural thickening, with infolding of a portion of the underlying lung. It is always situated adjacent to a pleural surface, with evidence of focal pleural thickening, particularly on CT scanning. Other causes of localized pleural thickening such as rheumatoid arthritis may cause rounded atelectasis, but asbestos-related disease is the most common cause in the United States.

Radiography. — A rounded opacity is present adjacent to a pleural surface, usually in the posterior and basal portion of a hemithorax. Evidence of pleural thickening is usually present. On tomography (conventional or CT), adjacent vessels will be distorted and deviated toward the mass, forming a "comet tail" sign.

When these signs are present, and percutaneous biopsy reveals no malignant cells, these patients may be followed without resorting to exploratory thoracotomy in every instance.

5) Malignant Mesothelioma

This malignant tumor has a well-known association with asbestos exposure. There is a latent period of over 30 years between the initial exposure and appearance of the tumor. Patients typically present with chest pain, weight loss, and variable degrees of dyspnea. Tumor bulk is often large at presentation, precluding curative resection. Histologic diagnosis often requires open, incisional biopsy as percutaneous needle biopsy is often falsely negative. In addition, differentiation between malignant mesothelioma and metastatic adenocarcinoma from an extrathoracic source is often difficult: both may present as diffuse pleural thickening with an associated pleural effusion. Differentiation is usually possible using a combination of electron microscopy and immunocytochemical studies.

Radiography. — The usual presentation of malignant mesothelioma is localized or diffuse pleural thickening, associated with a pleural effusion. If the effusion is large, the underlying pleural mass may not be visible. This tumor should be suspected whenever a large effusion is not associated with the expected shift of the mediastinum to the opposite side. Tumor mass often encases the lung, particularly on the mediastinal aspect, preventing mediastinal shift. Extensive encasement is most evident on thoracic CT, when differentiation between pleural fluid and tumor is easily accomplished. Pleural plaques, not visible on conventional radiography, may be seen on CT. Finally, the presence of rib destruction adjacent to the mass affords another clue to the correct diagnosis.

Asbestos-Related Parenchymal Abnormalities

Asbestos-Related Interstitial Fibrosis (Asbestosis)

The term "asbestosis" should be reserved for radiographically and/or histologically evident interstitial fibrosis known to be the result of asbestos exposure. The frequency of fibrosis is related to the magnitude and duration of exposure. Inhaled fibers penetrate the distal airways where a peribronchiolar fibrosis around the respiratory bronchioles is seen as the earliest histologic lesion. Initially there is predominant involvement of the lower lobes, with subsequent progression upward and toward the visceral pleural surface. With extensive fibrosis, the visceral pleural surface may be appreciably thickened.

Radiography.— The characteristic appearance of asbestosis is that of small, irregular shadows in the lower lungs. These shadows will increase in size and number (profusion) as more fibrosis ensues. In the standardized International Labor Office (ILO) classification and nomenclature, these opacities are called s, t and u opacities, corresponding to opacities demonstrated on standard radiographs provided by that organization for comparative and epidemiologic purposes. When extensive pleural and parenchymal fibrosis is present, the cardiac and hemidiaphragmatic margins appear "shaggy." Fibrosis within interlobular septa may give rise to septal (Kerley) lines. Cystic change, reflecting pathologic "honeycombing," may be evident in advanced cases. Asbestos does *not* produce the small, round opacities that are characteristic of silicosis and coal worker's pneumoconiosis.

Bronchogenic Carcinoma and Asbestos

Asbestos exposure is associated with an increased

risk of developing primary bronchogenic carcinoma. This risk is even further magnified in persons who smoke. Any histologic type of lung cancer may occur. Cancer should be suspected whenever a focal, localized opacity is present, and may have to be differentiated from rounded atelectasis.

Silicosis

This pneumoconiosis results from inhalation of crystalline silica (silicon dioxide), usually in the form of quartz. Significant amounts of silica may be inhaled during the mining of gold and other heavy metals, as the metal-bearing ores contain quartz. Other occupations that are associated with silica exposure include sandblasters in the ceramics and pottery industries, iron and steel foundry workers, and dental workers who use silica in the preparation of molds. Importantly, coal miners may inhale significant amounts of silica.

Pathology

Silica crystals that reach the alveoli are phagocytized by alveolar macrophages, which are subsequently recognized as "dust cells." Macrophage dissolution is followed by the release of soluble factors that promote the multiplication of fibroblasts and subsequent fibrosis. The classic histologic lesion is the "silicotic nodule," which is composed of concentric layers of collagen giving rise to an onion skin appearance. This accellular, collagenous nodule is quite different from the basic lesion resulting from coal exposure, to be described later.

The superimposition of many individual, subliminal nodules gives rise to the small, nodular shadows seen on chest radiography. The affected person is usually asymptomatic with this form of simple silicosis. However, continued exposure results in increasing fibrosis and loss of lung volume; small nodules will coalesce to form larger conglomerate masses (progressive massive fibrosis) about which areas of irregular emphysema appear. The patient may become severely disabled due to this form of complicated silicosis.

Radiography

Simple Silicosis.—The classic appearance is that of small, nodular shadows in the upper lung zones. The ILO nomenclature describes these shadows as p, q, and r opacities: p, up to 1.5 mm; q, 1.5 to 3 mm; r, 3 to 10 mm. The small, irregular shadows characteristic of asbestosis are *not* a feature of silicosis. Calcification within these nodules may be seen, but this is not common. Pleural disease is also not a feature of silicosis.

Complicated Silicosis.— With increasing fibrosis, coalescence of nodules occurs. The actual number of nodular shadows decreases as larger opacities (a large opacity is any nodular shadow larger than 1 cm) appear in the center of the upper lobes. Finally, large bilateral opacities may be present, simulating primary bronchogenic carcinomas. These large opacities may appear "thick" on one projection, but "thin" on the orthogonal projection, particularly on tomography. Clues to the correct diagnosis include the associated volume loss, irregular emphysema, and central migration of the opacities over time. An important associated feature is the frequent presence of lymph node enlargement with "egg-shell" calcification in the periphery of the node. Other rare causes of this pattern of lymph node calcification include amyloidosis and sarcoidosis. Whenever a diagnosis of complicated silicosis is made, comparison with previous radiographs should be made whenever possible. This is particularly important whenever there is clinical suspicion of lung cancer or reactivation tuberculosis.

Coal Worker's Pneumoconiosis

Inhalation of carbon in the form of coal has long been recognized as a cause of inorganic dust pneumoconiosis. However, coal miners frequently inhale significant amounts of silica contained in the surrounding ores. Thus, anthracosilicosis may be present, but is usually indistinguishable from "pure" coal worker's pneumoconiosis or "pure" silicosis.

Pathology

Inhaled carbon dust deposits preferentially around respiratory bronchioles, where the particles become enmeshed in a reticulin network. Microscopically, a central nidus of anthracotic pigment is surrounded by an irregular, dense collection of reticulin fibers and mild irregular emphysema. This "focal coal macule" is quite different from the silicotic nodule described earlier.

Radiography

The differentiation between simple and complicated coal worker's pneumoconiosis follows the same principles described for silicosis. Indeed, one may not be able to differentiate between the two conditions solely on the basis of the radiograph.

Unusual radiographic manifestations include cavitation of large opacities after spontaneous expectoration of a large amount of anthracotic material (this does not occur in complicated silicosis), and the coexistence of rheumatoid nodules in the same patient: Caplan's syndrome.

Berylliosis

This disorder is included in this section as it is an occupationally acquired disease, but its pathogenesis is very different from that of the other fibrogenic pneumoconioses.

Workers exposed to beryllium include those in the aerospace and electronic industries. This low atomic weight metal is alloyed with other metals to produce materials that are heat resistant, hard, and corrosion resistant. An acute, intense exposure to beryllium may result in acute lung injury with diffuse alveolar damage. Chronic, low-level exposure will result in interstitial lung disease.

Reaction to beryllium is systemic, and involves primarily a type IV immune response with granuloma formation. In this respect, it is very similar to sarcoidosis, which may also involve many organs. Pathologically, noncaseating granulomas are found, indistinguishable from those of sarcoidosis. It is prudent to consider berylliosis whenever a diagnosis of sarcoidosis is first made. This may be done by obtaining an occupational history and documenting in vitro transformation of sensitized T-lymphocytes on exposure to beryllium when this disease is suspected.

Radiography

In acute berylliosis, diffuse, bilateral consolidation may be seen. This primarily reflects increased permeability pulmonary edema, and diffuse alveolar damage.

Chronic berylliosis may present with small nodular and irregular shadows, simulating sarcoidosis and sometimes the other pneumoconioses such as asbestosis. Thoracic lymph node enlargement may be present. Calcification of parenchymal nodules may occur, but is rare. When extensive interstitial fibrosis is present, the appearance is indistinguishable from other known causes of parenchymal fibrosis.

HYPERSENSITIVITY PNEUMONITIS

This disease results from inhalation of organic dusts in the workplace or home. It is an immune-mediated disorder, also known as extrinsic allergic alveolitis. The number of occupations and hobbies associated with hypersensitivity pneumonitis is very large, but the most prevalent antigens and associated disorders in the United States are:

1. Thermophilic actinomycetes (fungal spores) (farmer's lung; ventilation pneumonitis); and
2. Avium serum proteins (bird-breeder's lung).

Pathogenesis

There is evidence that type III (immune complex) and type IV (cell-mediated) immune reactions are involved in hypersensitivity pneumonitis. Histologic examination in the setting of acute symptoms has revealed evidence of a pulmonary vasculitis, with deposition of immunoglobulins and C3 in and around affected vessels. Open lung biopsy later in the course of the disease reveals a granulomatous interstitial reaction, with prominent lymphocytic infiltration. Bronchoalveolar lavage yields abnormally high numbers of T-lymphocytes, particularly T-suppressor cells. If the disease is uncontrolled, progressive fibrosis ensues.

Clinical Presentation and Diagnosis

Patients may present with acute symptoms and signs such as dyspnea, nonproductive cough, fever, chills, and malaise. Typically, there is a latent period of 6 to 8 hours between the exposure and the onset of symptoms. Rales may be heard over the lower lungs. Precipitating antibodies to the offending antigen may be found in the serum, but these may also be present in exposed but unaffected persons. Thus, there is a definite individual susceptibility to this disease. In the chronic form, patients may present with marked weight loss and dyspnea due to pulmonary fibrosis.

The diagnosis may be made by a combination of clinical examination, radiography, and, most importantly, a history of exposure to an appropriate antigen. Open lung biopsy is rarely necessary.

Radiography

In the acute setting, there may be diffuse, small irregular and nodular shadows. However, the chest radiograph may be normal in spite of significant symptoms and abnormal pulmonary function tests. The finding of a normal radiograph in the presence of diffuse infiltrative disease demonstrated on lung biopsy has also been described with sarcoidosis, usual and desquamative interstitial pneumonia, and asbestosis.

With the development of interstitial fibrosis, small irregular shadows will increase in profusion, and cystic change, reflecting pathologic honeycombing, will appear. At this stage, the radiographic pattern may be indistinguishable from the many other causes of interstitial fibrosis.

SELECTED REFERENCES

Costabel U: The alveolitis of hypersensitivity pneumonitis. *Eur Respir J* 1988; 1:5.

Craighead JE, Mossman BT: The pathogenesis of asbestos-associated diseases. *N Engl J Med* 1982; 306:1446.

Gefter WB, Epstein DM, Miller WT: Radiographic evaluation of asbestos related chest disorders. *Crit Rev Diagn Imag* 1984; 21:133.

Kriebel D, Brain JD, Sprince NL, et al: The pulmonary toxicity of beryllium. *Am Rev Respir Dis* 1988; 137:464.

Morgan WKC, Lapp NL: Respiratory disease in coal miners. *Am Rev Respir Dis* 1976; 113:531.

Reynolds HY: Concepts of pathogenesis and lung reactivity in hypersensitivity pneumonitis. *Ann NY Acad Sci* 1986; 465:287.

Sargent EN, Lundell CJ: The pneumoconioses, in Taveras JM, Ferrucci JT (eds): *Radiology, Diagnosis-Imaging-Intervention*. Philadelphia, JB Lippincott Co, 1985, vol 1.

Ziskind M, Jones R, Weill H: Silicosis. *Am Rev Respir Dis* 1976; 113:643.

10

Pulmonary Vasculitis

Howard Mann, M.D.

KEY CONCEPTS

1. The pathogenesis of vasculitis involves immune complex formation and complement activation.
2. Deposition of immune complexes may result in "activation" of macrophages and T-lymphocytes, with subsequent granulomatous vasculitis.
3. Vascular occlusion is the end-result of vasculitis. Distal ischemia is associated with tissue necrosis.
4. Vasculitis involving postcapillary venules and capillaries in the lung results in interstitial and alveolar hemorrhage.
5. Vasculitic syndromes frequently involve the respiratory tract, skin, and kidneys concurrently.

The pulmonary vascular bed may be a specific site of injury in a wide variety of distinct vasculitic syndromes. These disorders are generally systemic, with the lung being only one of many organs involved in the disease process. The physiologic effects of involvement of extrapulmonary organs, such as the skin and kidney, usually dictate the clinical presentation, patient management, and prognosis. A specific histologic diagnosis is frequently made from renal or skin biopsies, and thus the opportunity to obtain radiologic-pathologic correlation related to lung involvement is limited.

The following discussion will include a set of definitions related to the pathology of vasculitis, a description of the pathogenesis of vasculitis, a classification scheme, and a description of the usual pulmonary radiographic manifestations of the various vasculitic syndromes.

PATHOLOGIC DEFINITIONS

The term vasculitis simply refers to the presence of an inflammatory process affecting the wall of a blood vessel. A typical histologic feature of this process is necrosis of the vascular wall with fibrin deposition, so-called fibrinoid necrosis. This is generally evident when the process affects medium- and large-sized arteries and veins. The end result is vascular occlusion and necrosis of tissue.

When the inflammatory process affects primarily postcapillary venules, a leukocytoclastic vasculitis is the histologic feature. This term describes the presence of abundant neutrophils and nuclear dust (from neutrophil death and degeneration) in and about the damaged blood vessels. This form of vasculitis is the basic lesion in the hypersensitivity vasculitides, which primarily involve the skin.

Capillaritis describes the presence of capillary disruption in association with intravascular and perivascular neutrophilic infiltration. In the lung, a frequent result of neutrophilic capillaritis is capillary and alveolar septal disruption with resultant interstitial and alveolar hemorrhage.

Granulomatous vasculitis refers to the presence of a granulomatous reaction involving the vessel wall. There is usually extensive necrosis, and the remnants of blood vessel wall elastic tissue may only be apparent with elastic stains. Palisading histiocytes and giant cells may be seen at the margin of the necrotic area, but sarcoid-like granulomas are not a feature.

In each specific vasculitic syndrome, there is predominant involvement of vessels of a particular size, and this is reflected in the characteristic clinical and radiographic presentation of each syndrome to be outlined in the classification scheme presented later.

PATHOGENETIC MECHANISMS IN VASCULITIS

It is generally accepted that the precipitating event leading to vasculitis is immune complex formation. In some conditions the antigen is known (e.g., streptococcal-associated glomerulonephritis, hepatitis B virus–associated vasculitis, and cryoprecipitable IgM/endogenous IgG in essential mixed cryoglobulinemia), but in most cases it is unknown. When immune complex formation occurs in the presence of slight antigen excess, the complexes lodge in blood vessel formation. Complement activation follows, with the generation of active complement factors such as C3a and C5a, which are chemoattractants for neutrophils. Neutrophil accumulation is followed by the release of neutrophil-derived proteases such as elastase, resulting in vascular inflammation and damage. The role of immune complexes is inferred from immunofluorescence studies that reveal granular deposits of IgG, IgM, the C3 component of complement and fibrinogen in vessel walls, and from electron microscopy studies that demonstrate subendothelial electron-dense deposits believed to represent immune complexes.

It is also accepted that immune complexes may precipitate granuloma formation. In the presence of slight antibody excess, deposition of immune complexes may occur. Recognition by "sensitized" macrophages and T-lymphocytes results in the production of interleukins 1 and 2, which result in the local accumulation and proliferation of additional activated T-lymphocytes. Specific sensitized T-lymphocytes also produce lymphokines, such as macrophage migration inhibitory factor and monocyte attractant factor. The result is granuloma formation, as monocytes leave the circulation to differentiate into tissue macrophages, which in turn serve as precursors of epithelioid and giant cells.

CLASSIFICATION OF THE VASCULITIC SYNDROMES

Many classification schemes have been proposed, all of which are somewhat arbitrary. The disorders listed in Table 10-1 include those that are usually described under the term "pulmonary angiitis and granulomatosis," such as Wegener's granulomatosis and the Churg-Strauss syndrome. Other disorders such as polyarteritis nodosa and temporal arteritis do not primarily affect the lung parenchyma. Importantly, patients may present with features of more than one of these distinct syndromes, with or without lung involvement. For example, a leukocytoclastic vasculitis involving the skin may accompany a medium-sized arteritis and aneurysm formation in the kidney. This pattern of involvement has been termed the "polyangiitis overlap syndrome."

Wegener's Granulomatosis

This disorder may occur in both children and adults, but the mean age at diagnosis is approximately 40 years. The disease is extremely rare in blacks. The principal pathologic finding is a necrotizing granulomatous vasculitis; both arteries and veins may be involved. In the classic form, there is involvement of the upper and lower respiratory tracts and kidneys. Patients may present with a wide variety of signs and symptoms such as chronic cough, chest pain, weight loss, malaise/fatigue, fever, arthralgias, sinus pain, and nasal discharge. A limited form of the disease involving only the lower respiratory tract at presentation may occur: pathergic Wegener's granulomatosis. Other organs that are not uncommonly involved are the skin, middle ear, and eye. A histologic diagnosis is usually made from a lung biopsy which will show characteristic granulomatous vasculitis and extravascular granulomas.

Sinus or nasopharyngeal biopsies are frequently nonspecific, as evidence of a vasculitis is commonly absent. It is important to make the diagnosis, as therapy

TABLE 10–1.
The Distinct Vasculitic Syndromes*

Vasculitic Syndrome	Vessels Involved	Pathologic Features	Distinctive Features
Polyarteritis nodosa	Small and medium-sized arteries	Necrotizing vasculitis	Angiographic evidence of aneurysms in renal, hepatic, and visceral vasculature
Allergic angiitis and granulomatosis (Churg-Strauss syndrome)	Small and medium-sized arteries	Granulomatous vasculitis	Allergic history, eosinophilia, pulmonary involvement
Hypersensitivity vasculitis	Arterioles, capillaries, venules, rarely small muscular arteries	Leukocytoclastic vasculitis	Skin involvement common, single type of vessel involvement usual
Henoch-Schönlein purpura	Venules, capillaries, arterioles	Leukocytoclastic vasculitis	Skin, gastrointestinal, renal involvement usual, IgA in immune complexes
Takayasu's arteritis	Medium-sized and large arteries	Giant cell arteritis	Predilection for aortic arch

Temporal arteritis	Medium-sized and large arteries	Giant cell arteritis	Predilection for branches of carotid
Wegener's granulomatosis	Small arteries and veins, medium-sized arteries	Necrotizing granulomatous vasculitis	Involvement of upper and lower respiratory tracts, glomerulonephritis common, varying degrees of small vessel vasculitis

*From Leavitt RY, Fauci AS: Polyangiitis overlap syndrome. *Am J Med* 1986; 81:79-85. Reproduced by permission.

with steroids and cyclophosphamide has well established efficacy.

Radiography

The usual presentation is that of localized parenchymal nodules of varying size. Cavitation within a large nodule or nodules due to tissue necrosis is a frequent occurrence, and air-fluid levels may be seen. A fluid level may also indicate the presence of bacterial superinfection within the cavity. The margins of the nodules may be sharply or poorly defined. The nodules may resolve to reappear in a different location. Pleural effusions and hilar lymph node enlargement are very uncommon. A rare presentation is localized or diffuse consolidation due to pulmonary hemorrhage, reflecting small vessel vasculitis or capillaritis.

Concurrent involvement of the upper respiratory tract usually manifests with mucosal thickening and variable opacification of the paranasal sinuses. Rarely, tracheal involvement may occur and result in diffuse segmental narrowing of the trachea.

Allergic Angiitis and Granulomatosis (Churg-Strauss Phenomenon)

This disease was originally described in patients with asthma and peripheral and tissue eosinophilia. The mean age at diagnosis is approximately 44 years, with a male-to-female ratio of 1.3:1. There is frequent involvement of other organs such as the skin and gastrointestinal tract by leukocytoclastic vasculitis. Clinically significant renal disease is not a common feature. The common occurrence of pulmonary disease serves to distinguish this disorder from polyarteritis nodosa. Pathologically, both vascular and extravascular granulomas may be found, similar to the findings in Wegener's granulomatosis. This also serves to differentiate this disorder from other causes of pulmonary opacities with eosinophilia such as Löffler's syndrome, parasitic infestation of the lung (tropical eosinophilia), and chronic eosinophilic pneumonia. Marked tissue eosinophilia is not a feature of Wegener's granulomatosis. However, it should be noted that the reference to allergy in the initial description of this disease was based on clinical and historical evidence of atopy, and not specific histologic findings per se. Thus, the presence of asthma and eosinophilia is perhaps more appropriately termed the Churg-Strauss phenomenon.

Radiography

Localized, nonsegmental parenchymal opacities are generally present. These are usually poorly marginated, and cavitation is rare. Opacities may resolve spontaneously. Pleural effusions may occur.

Polyarteritis Nodosa

This disease affects small- and medium-sized visceral arteries. Aneurysm formation is a typical result. However, granulomatous vasculitis is not a feature of this condition. In many patients, glomerulonephritis occurs, with focal necrosis and crescent formation. This pattern of vasculitis may occur as a result of hepatitis B virus infection, and may occasionally be seen in systemic lupus erythematosus (SLE), rheumatoid arthritis, and in approximately 30% of patients with hairy cell leukemia. Thus, polyarteritis nodosa may not be a specific pathologic entity. If pulmonary involvement and/or extravascular granulomas are present on biopsy, a different diagnosis should be considered, such as limited Wegener's granulomatosis or the polyangiitis overlap syndrome.

Hypersensitivity Vasculitis

This term applies to a heterogeneous group of disorders in which the inciting antigen may be an infectious agent (e.g., streptococci and hepatitis B virus), a drug, an endogenous antigen (e.g., native deoxyribonucleic acid in SLE), or a tumor-derived antigen (e.g., in paraneoplastic vasculitis). However, in most cases the offending antigen is unknown. Leukocytoclastic vasculitis typically affects the skin, manifesting as palpable purpura.

Hypersensitivity vasculitis is found in Henoch-Schönlein purpura, which usually occurs in the pediatric age group. The antibody involved in the immune complex reaction is IgA. Skin, renal, and gastrointestinal tract involvement is common, with the lungs only very rarely affected. Lung involvement takes the form of pulmonary hemorrhage, presumably due to a capillaritis.

Pulmonary involvement may also occur in a rare disorder hypocomplementemic urticarial vasculitis. Patients with this disorder may have clinical manifestations of obstructive airways disease in addition to characteristic urticarial skin lesions. It has been postulated that neutrophil accumulation following immune complex deposition results in the release of large amounts of neutrophil-derived elastase. Progressive destruction of alveolar walls leads to macroscopic emphysema.

Temporal Arteritis

This form of giant cell arteritis primarily affects branches of the external carotid artery. The diagnosis is made on biopsy of the temporal artery, and the disease responds to steroid therapy. Pulmonary involvement is not a feature.

Takayasu's Arteritis

This disease classically affects the aorta and its major branches. The end result is vascular narrowing and occlusion; hence the term "pulseless disease." Importantly, involvement of the large pulmonary arteries may occur, with vascular stenoses and occlusion evident on angiography. Symptomatic pulmonary hypertension may result. Histologic confirmation is not usually required, but if biopsy specimens are obtained, an arteritis with mononuclear cell infiltration and giant cells will be seen.

Immune Complex Disease and Vasculitis in Other Disorders

Immune complex deposition and resultant vasculitis has been described in a diverse group of diseases not encompassed within the spectrum of distinct vasculitic syndromes described. Symptomatic pulmonary involvement in these diseases is relatively uncommon. The frequency of pathologic pulmonary disease is unknown, primarily because lung biopsies are rarely obtained.

Pulmonary vasculitis has been found pathologically in the following disorders:

1. Systemic lupus erythematosus;
2. Rheumatoid arthritis/Sjögren's syndrome;
3. Essential mixed cryoglobulinemia;
4. Behçet's syndrome;
5. Nodular (necrotizing) sarcoidosis;
6. Idiopathic crescentic glomerulonephritis with systemic vasculitis; and
7. Infections, particularly from fungal/mycobacterial organisms.

RADIOLOGIC-PATHOLOGIC CORRELATION

Localized or diffuse consolidation resulting from pulmonary hemorrhage may be seen. In most cases, pulmonary capillaritis is the presumed pathologic substrate. This is particularly the case in systemic lupus erythematosis and idiopathic crescentic glomerulonephritis with systemic vasculitis.

In Behçet's disease, involvement of large pulmonary arteries may result in in situ thrombosis and aneurysm formation. Pulmonary hemorrhage and infarction are well-recognized sequelae.

Vasculitis is a prominent pathologic feature in nodular sarcoidosis. Well-defined parenchymal nodules mimicking metastatic disease is the typical presentation. Hilar and mediastinal lymph node enlargement may or may not be present. In other respects, the disease is similar to classic sarcoidosis.

The radiographic findings in fungal and mycobacterial infections have been described previously. Pathologically, a prominent vasculitis may accompany granuloma formation, simulating Wegener's granulomatosis. The latter diagnosis should only be definitively made after studies with special stains to exclude fungal/mycobacterial organisms have been performed.

SELECTED REFERENCES

Falk DK: Pulmonary disease in idiopathic urticarial vasculitis. *J Am Acad Dermatol* 1984; 11:346.

Gamble CN, Wiesner KB, Shapiro RF: The immune complex pathogenesis of glomerulonephritis and pulmonary vasculitis in Behçet's disease. *Am J Med* 1979; 66:1031.

Leathermann JW, Davies SF, Hoidal JR: Alveolar hemorrhage syndromes: Diffuse microvascular lung hemorrhage in immune and idiopathic disorders. *Medicine* 1984; 63:343.

Leavitt RY, Fauci AS: Pulmonary vasculitis. *Am Rev Respir Dis* 1986; 134:149.

Leavitt RY, Fauci AS: Polyangiitis overlap syndrome. *Am J Med* 1985; 81:79.

Mark EJ, Ramirez JF: Pulmonary capillaritis and hemorrhage in patients with systemic vasculitis. *Arch Pathol Lab Med* 1985; 109:413.

McCluskey RT, Fienberg R: Vasculitis in primary vasculitides, granulomatoses and connective tissue diseases. *Hum Pathol* 1983; 14:305.

Sams WM, Thorne EG, Small P, et al: Leukocytoclastic vasculitis. *Arch Dermatol* 1976; 112:219.

11

Lung Injury

David G. Bragg, M.D.

KEY CONCEPTS

1. Appropriate radiographic screening for rib fractures can be accomplished with a routine chest x-ray.
2. Flail chest segment—three or more contiguous segmental rib fractures.
3. High rib fractures suggest mediastinal injury with lower (caudal) fractures—visceral (liver, spleen) injury.
4. A pleural air-fluid level *always* indicates a pneumothorax.
5. Lung parenchymal injuries include contusion (appears immediately/resolves quickly), and laceration.
6. Traumatic aortic lacerations occur near the ligamentum arteriosum and can only be detected by angiography.
7. Radiation lung injury, acute and chronic, can be confidently characterized by chest x-ray. The "rule of sixes" can be used to recall the time frames.
8. Drug injury to the lung is usually reflected by a diffuse, nonspecific interstitial infiltrate.

PENETRATING TRAUMA

The imaging requirements for the patient with penetrating chest trauma are usually obvious, as the patient most often presents with a known injury. The role of the radiologist should focus on the following questions:

- Is there a pneumothorax?
- Is there evidence of a foreign body?
- Is there evidence of fluid (blood) in the pleural compartment?
- Is there mediastinal emphysema?
- Is the mediastinal contour obscured or widened?
- Is the cardiac contour normal, enlarged or obscured?

The nature and extent of penetrating lung injuries relate to the weapon or object employed in the generation of the injury. Knife wounds may leave a very small point of entry yet be responsible for major injury to the pleura, lung parenchyma, and vascular structures. The radiologist should know the point of entry and—if one is present—the exit site. The type of missile or object used in the trauma should also be known to adequately define the extent of injury as well as the presence or absence of a foreign body.

The abnormalities that relate to the pleura, mediastinum, and heart will be discussed in greater detail in the section that follows.

BLUNT CHEST TRAUMA

General Features

The manifestations of blunt chest trauma are primarily those resulting from auto/pedestrian injuries. In these instances, rapid deceleration and direct external forces applied to the chest result in significant injuries to the chest wall, lung, and mediastinal contents. The initial chest x-ray provides the most specific information as to the extent of this injury, which is often not evident on physical examination. Each of the thoracic compartments should be assessed independently to evaluate the total extent of the injuries. Occasionally, the findings may be complex or confusing due to injury of a pre-existing condition such as the rupture of a bulla, an underlying clotting disorder, or pre-existing cardiac or mediastinal abnormality.

As summarized in the section on penetrating trauma, specific history and symptoms related by the patient should be known to the radiologist at the time of the review of the chest x-ray. Any questions or concerns should lead to examination of the patient and evaluation of specific clinical findings.

Chest Wall

Injuries to the thoracic cage are expressed differently in the younger patient than in the older individual. The rigidity of the thoracic cage in the older individual exposed to significant blunt trauma almost invariably causes fractures, with obvious displacement of the opposed rib segments. In contrast, the more compliant chest wall of the younger individual either may not fracture in spite of significant intrathoracic injury, or the fracture may be so minimally displaced as to not be evident on the chest x-ray. In either instance, the routine posteroanterior and lateral chest x-ray is an adequate screening measure for the detection of either displaced rib segments or as baseline measure to evaluate soft tissue injury to the pleura, parenchyma, or mediastinal contents. Should the rib be fractured, but not displaced, the x-ray beam may not traverse the fracture line, hence making the fracture invisible. This oversight is not clinically significant as the patient's treatment will not be materially affected. Specific rib detail films are only of interest in further evaluating rib trauma or in the assessment of a possible flail-chest segment. This latter injury is a segmental fracture of three or more contiguous ribs, anteriorly and posteriorly. This anatomic segment may be of sufficient size to be physiologically significant (paradoxical motion) with the ventilatory dynamics of the lung. If obvious fractures are evident, one should carefully inspect the ribs to be certain whether or not three or more segmental, contiguous rib fractures are present to qualify as a flail-chest type of injury.

Fractures of lower ribs are much more frequently associated with visceral injury to either the liver, spleen, or kidneys. Fractures involving the lower ribs should draw the radiologist's attention to these visceral organs as possible sites for occult injury. Fractures of the more cranial ribs were earlier felt to be predictors for major vessel injury, including the aorta and great vessels as well as the tracheobronchial area. Subsequent reports have indicated that such fractures have low predictive value for such injuries.

Subcutaneous emphysema following blunt chest trauma is usually a predictor of pleural laceration. Subcutaneous emphysema may occasionally follow mediastinal emphysema, without pleural tear/pneumothorax being present. The emphysema camouflages the chest so that underlying lung injury may be difficult to recognize. One should assume that a pneumothorax is present when subcutaneous emphysema is observed. Also, one should carefully evaluate the thoracic cage, particularly in its posterior-lateral region to look for the often subtle, minimally displaced rib fractures.

Pleura

The individual involved in multiple trauma must usually be evaluated with supine or semierect portable chest radiographs. The technical compromises associated with the supine portable technique limit the ability to detect a small pneumothorax. As mentioned earlier, overlying subcutaneous emphysema may be present which further restricts the observer's ability to visualize the thin pleural line of the collapsed lung. With the patient in the recumbent position, the pneumothorax is usually best visualized laterally in contrast to its apical location on the erect chest x-ray. It is not necessary to judge the percentage of the pneumothorax, an estimate that is fraught with interobserver variation. One may use approximations as to the volume of the hemithorax to give gross estimations as to the percent of the pneumothorax.

Initially, any fluid present in the pleural cavity can be assumed to represent blood. Occasionally, on the erect chest x-ray, a stright fluid level will be observed at the base of the lung even though a pleural edge representing a pneumothorax may not be visible. Whenever a straight air-fluid level is observed within the pleural compartment, a hydropneumothorax is present.

Lung Parenchyma

Three types of blunt traumatic lung parenchymal injury may occur: contusion and two laceration subtypes (pneumatocele and hematoma).

Contusion

A lung contusion is visible on the chest x-ray as an air space or alveolar infiltrate, peripherally oriented in either a lobar or segmental distribution. This peripheral location and immediate presentation is followed by a rapid radiographic resolution, as the lung serves as a very efficient absorber of blood. The contusion should have disappeared in 48 to 72 hours.

Laceration

A lung laceration is a fracture of a group of secondary pulmonary lobules contained and made spherical by the inflationary pressures of the surrounding lung. The appearance of these lacerations on the chest x-ray is determined by whether an adjacent blood vessel has also been lacerated and/or a communication with a bronchus exists. There are therefore two subtypes of lung lacerations based upon these associated factors:

Pneumatocele (Traumatic Lung Cyst).— A pneumatocele is a simple laceration of a cluster of secondary pulmonary lobules without involving a blood vessel. It is a well-defined spherical air cyst on the chest x-ray. This traumatic pneumatocele is often camouflaged by the surrounding lung contusion and does not become evident until later x-ray (2 to 3 days following injury), when the contusion has resolved.

Hematoma.— A hematoma is a water-density

spherical "nodule" which resembles the lung cyst or pneumatocele except that a vessel has been lacerated along with the secondary pulmonary lobules. The lung cyst therefore fills with blood or forms an air fluid level if a communication with a bronchus exists. According to Fagan and Ellis (see Selected References), it takes much longer for this type of a lesion to resolve than the simple pneumatocele, usually months in contrast to the weeks required for a simple pneumatocele.

Mediastinum

Tracheobronchial Fracture

Fractures of the tracheobronchial tree are uncommon injuries resulting from rapid deceleration and are limited to the distal trachea and proximal 1 to 2 cm of the bronchus. Radiographic signs suggesting laceration of the tracheobronchial tree on initial films include a medial pneumothorax, mediastinal and "deep" cervical emphysema (emphysema confined to the deep cervical fascial planes), or fractures of ribs one through three. Later a persistent pneumothorax and atelectasis in spite of chest tube placement should suggest the need for endoscopy to further evaluate the possibility of a tracheobronchial laceration. Uncommonly, the collapsed lung may "drop" or at least change its position when the patient is moved from a recumbent to an erect projection, reflecting the loss of the tethering effect of the intact bronchus.

According to Harvey-Smith et al., bronchial fractures are associated with a high mortality (approximating 30%), and with significant morbidity, as the definitive diagnosis is usually delayed.

Heart

Injuries to the heart following blunt chest trauma are usually radiographically occult. The most common form of injury is merely a mild cardiac contusion which usually is not associated with any radiographic abnormality. The patient will complain of discomfort and signs suggesting a pericarditis, often with abnormalities on the electrocardiogram. One can assume the presence of underlying cardiac injury in individuals with sternal fractures, as they are virtually always associated with underlying cardiac trauma, usually contusion.

The more serious cardiac injuries are much less frequent and involve lacerations of the septal walls, usually the interventricular septum. Traumatic injury to the valves most frequently involve either the aortic or mitral valves. These injuries may be evident immediately or be delayed by some days or weeks, with the individual presenting with cardiac symptoms, an enlarged heart with or without evidence of heart failure, and new murmur.

Traumatic Aortic Laceration

A critical decision pathway must be chosen in the individual with significant chest trauma who has an abnormal mediastinum on chest x-ray. This decision relates to the possibility of traumatic rupture of the aorta, an injury which accounts for nearly 16% of fatalities resulting from motor vehicle accidents at present. Most of these injuries are responsible for the patient's immediate death, as a transmural laceration of the aorta is invariably fatal. Patients with aortic laceration who survive to reach a hospital are the ones who require critical evaluation and a decision regarding the need for thoracic aortography. These are lesions in which a deceleration type of trauma lacerates the aorta at the level of the ligamentum arteriosum. This structure is at the distal portion of the aortic arch and acts to anchor the aorta as the rest of the great vessel proximal and distal to this point continue to accelerate, fracturing the wall of the aorta and leading to the laceration and traumatic dissecting aneurysm.

Aortography with contrast medium is the only definitive diagnostic procedure available to detect and define a traumatic aortic dissection or laceration. In a critically injured patient, a decision to proceed to aortography should be based on the clinical situation and plain film observations. An attempt should be made to obtain a "true" erect chest radiograph, usually limited to portable technique. Only a normal chest x-ray is a useful predictor to exclude the presence of an aortic laceration. Multiple plain film findings have been described in association with traumatic aortic rupture, all related to the non-specific presence of mediastinal hemorrhage (nasogastric tube placement, depression of the left main stem bronchus, obscuration of the aortic contour, mediastinal widening, pleural fluid, left paraspinal stripe widening, high rib fractures, and so forth). None of these individual observations is sufficiently sensitive (9% to 12% in a report by Mirvis et al.) to accurately establish a plain film diagnosis. The decision to proceed to aortography should therefore be based on the clinical likelihood of aortic injury combined with the presence or absence of plain film abnormalities; the more present, the greater their cumulative predictive value.

The strategy is to recognize the predictive values of these radiologic plain film findings, combine them with the clinical probability of a dissection being present, and proceed with a contrast-material injection of the aorta, either using digital subtraction angiography or routine thoracic aortography. It has been suggested by Mirvis et al. that computed tomography (CT) and magnetic resonance imagery may obviate the need for aortography; however, greater experience with these techniques is needed to recommend their use in the routine setting.

Diaphragmatic Rupture

Traumatic rupture of the hemidiaphragm is an uncommon consequence of blunt chest trauma which often is detected sometime after the initial injury. Earlier reports suggested that the injury was almost invariably left-sided; however, more recent reports have shown a nearly equal frequency of right and left diaphragmatic injuries. The location of the injury will obviously alter the plain film finding as with right-sided injury; displacement of the liver is the result whereas bowel contents are usually displaced into the chest with left-sided injuries. In nearly one quarter of the patients, the chest x-ray will show no abnormalities to suggest a diaphragmatic rupture.

With left-sided laceration, the stomach is the most common organ displaced into the hemithorax. As multiple other injuries usually are present in association with a diaphragmatic laceration, the diagnosis is often overlooked. If one suspects a diaphragmatic laceration on the left side, a nasogastric tube should be inserted into the stomach, and its course high in the left hemithorax should suggest the diagnosis. Contrast material will usually not be necessary unless, in the less common late presentation of diaphragmatic rupture, the left colon is found to be in the thorax, which will require a contrast enema to confirm the diagnosis.

If a right-sided injury is present, a radionuclide liver-spleen scan will confirm the diagnosis. CT scans are now the more frequent confirmatory techniques utilized (see references by Heiberg et al. and Waldschmidt et al.) even though the challenge may be significant to both detect the site of the laceration and make the correct diagnosis.

RADIATION INJURY

The effects of radiation on the lung have been recognized for over 60 years. Unfortunately, problems in terminology have mistakenly identified radiation changes as "pneumonitis." There is virtually no inflammatory component to the process which is better referred to as "radiation change or injury."

Pathology

Histologic findings in radiation injury are nonspecific and vary with time following the completion of radiation. Within the first 6 months, the acute phase is characterized by endothelial injury. The endothelial cells become swollen with cell degeneration and sloughing as well as capillary injury, causing an abnormal accumulation of cell debris and plasma which floods the alveolar compartment within the area of the radiation port. The later changes are almost entirely interstitial and relate to thickening of the alveolar septa and hyaline membranes with retraction and volume loss. The pleural compartment may be affected during the first posttreatment year, resulting in a transudative effusion which spontaneously disappears. Small, clinically insignificant effusions may be noted in approximately 10% of patients following extensive thoracic radiation treatments. Later, pleural fibrosis and thickening, usually over the apex of the lung may be observed.

Clinical Course

The clinical course of radiation lung injury is related to the radiation dose, dose fractionation, the volume of lung treated, and any adjuvant therapy such as cytotoxic drugs and cortisone. The threshold for lung injury varies with the age of the patient and, occasionally, the disease. With conventional fractionation (150 to 200 rads) radiation injury to the lung will be noted with increasing frequency in patients receiving over 2,000 to 3,000 rads (20–30 Gy). The majority of patients will exhibit clinical and/or radiographic evidence of radiation injury with doses in excess of 5,000 rads (50 Gy). The latent period from treatment to clinical and/or radiographic evidence of injury decreases with increasing total dose, increasing fractionation (radiation dose per treatment) and increasing port size.

Certain cytotoxic drugs enhance the changes of radiation injury and may make their clinical and radiographic patterns different or atypical. The most important drug to understand is cortisone. When cortisone is cycled or withdrawn in a patient who has received pulmonary radiation therapy, a "recall" radiation injury may be noted sometime following the completion of the course of treatment. This "recall" injury mimics the typical clinical and radiographic injury but differs in developing some time following the completion of treatment, occasionally confusing the diagnosis.

Radiographic Course

To remember the time course associated with radiation injury, one should recall the "Rule of Sixes." This rule suggests that acute radiation injury should be evident within 6 weeks to 6 months following the completion of the course of radiation to the chest. Late radiation changes should be stable within 16 months following the completion of radiation therapy.

Acute Changes

Acute radiation changes again vary with the radiation dose, port size and location, patient age, and fractionation schedule. The acute radiation injury is characterized by air-space disease sharply contoured by the port. Now that tailored ports are used more frequently than the rectangular or square ports in years past, the margins of the radiation injury seen in the acute phase may be difficult to recognize and distinguish from anatomic landmarks. One should attempt to become familiar with the patient's history of radiation and also, be familiar with the radiation ports used in the individual's treatment to better understand and predict the nature of the radiation injury. The characteristic changes, however, are air-space disease which is port limited and pursues the predictable time period of 6 weeks to 6 months following the completion of treatment. Patient symptoms of a dry cough and occasionally, dyspnea with a low-grade fever are usually as nonspecific, as are the histologic changes. The radiographic diagnosis should be more obvious, particularly with knowledge of the radiation treatment regimen.

Chronic Changes

The chronic changes may or may not be heralded by the above described acute changes. The more dramatic the acute radiation injury, the more likely the chronic or late changes are to develop subsequently. These late changes are interstitial and associated with volume loss and retraction in contrast to the airspace characteristics of the acute injury. Again, the changes are port limited and are manifest by retraction, volume loss, stringy reticular infiltrates, and, occasionally, contiguous pleural thickening. The hilus is usually made less distinct and elevated cranially and the mediastinal margins are less distinct than normal.

The more common port designs used in the treatment of intrathoracic diseases are those associated with the treatment of breast cancer, Hodgkin's disease, and primary lung cancer. One should understand the design of the ports to be able to more easily predict the patterns of acute and late radiation changes seen on the chest radiography. In each of these diseases, the total dose used will exceed 4,500 rads (45 Gy), meaning that virtually all of these patients will have some radiation changes evident on routine chest x-rays. The individual treated for head and neck cancers also will have radiation change evident in the apices of the lung as the ports used invariably include that area to a dose in excess of 5,000 rads (50 Gy).

CT scanning is a more sensitive technique to detect radiation injury both in its acute and late forms. The changes are similar although more dramatic than those described above for routine chest x-ray findings. The port margins are more clearly defined by CT; however, the same general time frames, patterns of involvement and characteristics should apply. The only difference between CT and routine chest x-rays will be the greater sensitivity of CT in recognizing and specifically characterizing radiation lung injury.

DRUG INJURY

Drug-induced lung injury is now a large, complex, and growing problem which has assumed greater importance with the more potent and numerous agents used in clinical medicine. Organizationally, one should understand the types of adverse drug reactions and divide them into:

1. Drug overdose;
2. Understood side effects;
3. Secondary drug effects (e.g., immune suppression by steroids when given for arthritis);
4. Drug interactions (combination of drugs which enhance or inhibit each other);
5. Intolerance (an undesirable effect of the drug which is a normal pharmacologic response affecting the patient's ability to tolerate the agent); and/or
6. Idiosyncrasy (an untoward drug reaction which is not a normal pharmacologic action)
7. Hypersensitivity

In Table 11-1 the types of radiographic abnormalities are summarized by broad categories, some of the major clinical features, course and the more common drugs implicated in the process. By far the most common type of drug injury reflected on the chest x-ray is interstitial fibrosis, which usually results from the use of cancer chemotherapeutic agents. The patterns of disease are nonspecific and usually involve the lung base without other components of the thorax involved.

The mechanism of lung injury responsible for interstitial lung disease is poorly understood. The pathology is usually reflected by diffuse alveolar damage with an interstitial cellular infiltrate. The symptoms are nonspecific, and include dyspnea, cough, low-grade fever with a reduction in diffusing capacity and lung volumes on pulmonary function studies.

The chest radiographic patterns of pulmonary fibrosis due to drugs vary from normal to a nonspecific predominantly basilar pattern of interstitial fibrosis. Pleural effusions are uncommon and, unless other drugs are utilized, other anatomic compartments of the thorax are usually not involved. A notable exception is the striking skeletal deossification associated with the long-term administration of corticosteroids.

TABLE 11–1.
Drug-induced Chest Abnormalities

Types of Radiographic Abnormalities	Clinical Features	Reversibility	Drugs Implicated
Pleural-pericardial effusions	Shortness of breath SLE-like symptoms	Yes, upon drug withdrawal	Procainamide (Pronestyl) hydralazine, isoniazid, diphenylhydantoin methysergide
Alveolar infiltrates (hypersensitivity)	Acute shortness of breath Low-grade fever	Yes, upon drug withdrawal	Nitrofurantoin, methotrexate, procarbazine, cyclophosphamide, cytosine arabinoside, sulfas, penicillin, ampicillin, PAS, hydralazine, isoniazid
Interstial fibrosis	Dyspnea Cough Fatigue Malaise	Variable (some are steroid and drug withdrawal-responsive; others are progressive)	Cytotoxic agents, opiates, pituitary snuff, salicylates, methysergide, amiodarone

Lymph node enlargement	Usually none other than gum hypertrophy and palpable adenopathy	Usually regresses	Diphenylhydantoin, carbamazepine
Skeletal deossification	Pain with spontaneous fractures	Improves with drug withdrawal	Corticosteroids

Exceptions to this nonspecific pattern of diffuse pulmonary fibrosis may be seen with certain cytotoxic agents. Bleomycin causes nodular lesions more readily apparent on CT scans, which may mimic metastatic disease to the lung. Methotrexate originally was described as occurring in patients in remission from their acute leukemia who developed a clinical pattern resembling pneumocystis carinii pneumonia, with an acute onset of shortness of breath, dyspnea, cough, and low-grade fever. The chest x-ray abnormalities were a "ground-glass" chest x-ray pattern, occasionally with small pleural effusions. These infiltrates could be patchy or resemble pulmonary edema. The infiltrates tended to disappear upon drug withdrawal. A similar syndrome may occur in individuals treated with methotrexate for benign diseases including rheumatoid arthritis and psoriasis.

Most cytotoxic drugs do not appear to show a close association between cumulative drug dose and pulmonary toxicity. One exception is busulfan in which pulmonary damage may be expected to occur above a dose level of 500 mg. There was a less direct association with bleomycin where pulmonary toxicity seems to increase with cumulative doses above 450 to 500 units. Certainly, it has been shown that cardiac toxicity is closely related to the dose of adriamycin.

Treatment of lung disease due to cytotoxic agents is variable. In each instance, withdrawal of the drug should be the initial therapeutic measure, in most cases followed by a course of corticosteroids. In most of these patients, irreversible damage has already occurred to the lung.

The alveolar infiltrative abnormalities noted on the chest radiograph tend to reflect more acute, hypersensitivity reactions. A long list of drugs can be found responsible for the hypersensitivity types of lung injuries summarized in Table 11-1. The clinical symptoms are similar, usually with dyspnea and low-grade fever. The patchy, alveolar infiltrates are nonspecific and mimic infection or noncardiogenic pulmonary edema and are more acute and dramatic in onset than the more frequently observed interstitial changes, described earlier. Rarely, drugs may induce a form of bronchiolitis obliterans. This usually causes a focal pneumonic infiltrate in a single or cluster of areas in the lung. Bronchiolitis obliterans, organizing pneumonia is responsive to drug withdrawal and corticosteroids in the majority of cases, even though some may have a progressive course in fatal outcome.

Mediastinal lymph node enlargement has been reported in a small percentage of patients treated with anticonvulsant therapy, usually with diphenylhydantoin and carbamazepine. Usually, the lymph node enlargement follows long term drug administration and occasionally is associated with interstitial lung disease. The nodal enlargement responds to drug withdrawal alone in the majority of the cases, even though corticosteroids are often included in the treatment regimen.

Serous effusions may be associated with a lupus-like syndrome associated with a variety of pharmacologic agents. These drugs cause shortness of breath and lupus-like symptoms which usually disappear upon drug withdrawal. Pleural effusions and cardiac enlargement due to pericardial effusion may mimic the radiographic and clinical changes associated with heart failure adding further confusion as this is often the clinical condition for which the drugs causing this syndrome are prescribed.

Skeletal deossification has a unique association with corticosteroids. The diffuse skeletal deossification follows high-dose and long-term administration of steroids and may be associated with spontaneous rib and vertebral body fractures.

A very complete discussion of drug-induced pulmonary disease can be found in a two-part article (which is exhaustively referenced) by Cooper, White, and Matthay that appeared in the *American Review of Respiratory Diseases* in 1986 (133:321–340 and 133:488–505).

INHALATIONAL INJURIES

Respiratory complications from the inhalation of noxious gases occur primarily from smoke inhalation. Chemical compounds which are inhaled usually result from industrial accidents, with the agent known at the time the patient presents for the initial chest x-ray.

Noxious Gases and Aerosol Exposure

The clinical and radiographic patterns of chemical exposure are related to the agent, its concentration, and the duration of exposure. The more soluble the agent, the more likely the irritation will be limited to the external mucus membrane and upper airways (sulfur dioxide, ammonia, and chlorine). The less soluble agents (phosgene, nitrogen dioxide, ozone) cause injury to the distal portion of the airways, usually at the alveolo-capillary region. A later onset of injury may characterize the course of the patient exposed to noxious agents, which is the subsequent development of bronchiolitis obliterans, organizing pneumonia, some weeks following the initial exposure. Certain toxic materials such as the aromatic hydrocarbons reach the lung after being ingested, causing injury to the alveolo-capillary membrane. The example is best illustrated by the child who ingests hydrocarbons and subsequently develops a pneumonia without historical evidence of aspiration.

Smog contains a variety of ingredients, most notably ozone and nitrogen dioxide. Patient symptoms are far more common that radiographic abnormalities. Nitrogen dioxide is the causative agent in silo-filler's disease (farmer's lung). In this entity, nitrogen dioxide accumulates in an enclosed space housing silage, causing lung injury with significant exposure. Immediately after exposure, noncardiogenic pulmonary edema develops, which rapidly clears. Bronchiolitis obliterans may later develop in a small percentage of these individuals. Uncommonly, sulfur dioxide and ammonia may cause either bronchiolitis obliterans or bronchiectasis.

Carbon monoxide exposure has been associated with peripheral ground-glass infiltrates, probably representing edema from the direct effects of the gas on the alveolo-capillary membrane.

Smoke Inhalation

Respiratory complications from smoke inhalation are more important problems in the burn patient than thermal injury. Often, the smoke is combined with noxious gases so that a combination of injuries results, some of which have been described. The noxious gases in smoke combine with the atmospheric moisture and normal water in the lung to form corrosive acids and alkalis, occasionally causing direct chemical injury to the respiratory tract and also damage to the lupus alveolo-capillary membrane. The smoke will often cause a chemical tracheobronchitis, which is a leading clinical symptom upon initial presentation. An elevated carboxyhemoglobin level may also be noted to document the clinical problem.

The chest x-ray may be entirely normal on initial presentation; however, in many patients, nonspecific changes of peribronchial cuffing, perivascular fuzziness, or changes of alveolar-interstitial edema may be noted. The most specific imaging technique to make the diagnosis of smoke inhalational injury damage is done with xenon-133 ventilation lung scanning. This agent will show areas of ventilation-deficient zones in the lung, probably as a result of atelectasis and small airway obstruction due to the injury from the smoke. Patients exposed to noxious gases and smoke should have a baseline chest radiograph, with the realization that the chest x-ray is not a good predictor for underlying injury but nonetheless helps to anticipate many of the subsequent complications and certainly serves as a valid baseline.

Thermal Injury

Burns of the respiratory tree are usually limited to the oropharyngeal region and proximal trachea. Steam burns are usually more serious and disabling than those resulting from dry, hot air. Some clinicians even wonder whether or not thermal injury per se can occur below the level of the carina, as the upper respiratory tract is such an efficient heat exchanger, covered with moist mucosa. As an operational axiom, one should presume that lung injury in a burn patient has resulted from smoke and/or noxious gases rather than from thermal injury. These chemical or thermal injuries should be evident clinically and radiographically within 24 hours subsequent to exposure. Radiographic changes after that time usually are a reflection of the patient's state of hydration. Chest radiographic abnormalities other than those related to fluid status changes usually represent pneumonias. Initially (during the first 2 weeks following the injury) the infectious agents are pyogenic and later, after 2 to 3 weeks, fungal.

SELECTED REFERENCES

Ellis R: Traumatic lung cysts. *JAMA* 1976; 236:1976-1977.

Fagan CJ: Traumatic lung cysts. *AJR* 1966; 97:186-194.

Fagan CJ, Swischuk LE: Traumatic lung and paramediastinal pneumoathoceles. *Radiology* 1976; 120:11-18.

Harvey-Smith W, Bush W, Northrop C: Traumatic bronchial rupture. *AJR* 1980; 134:1189-1193.

Heiberg E, Wolverson MK, Hurd RN: CT recognition of traumatic rupture of the diaphragm. *AJR* 1980; 135:369-372.

Mirvis SE, Bidwell JK, Buddemeyer EU: Imaging diagnosis of traumatic aortic rupture: A review and experience at a major trauma center. *Invest Radiol* 1987; 2:187-196.

Waldschmidt BL, Laws HL: Injuries of the diaphragm. *J Trauma* 1980; 20:587-592.

RECOMMENDED ADDITIONAL READINGS

Ayella RJ: *Radiologic Management of the Massively Traumatized Patient*. Baltimore, Williams & Wilkins, 1978.

Belamy EA, Husband JE, Blaquiere RM, et al: Bleomycin-related lung damage: CT evidence. *Radiology* 1985; 156:155-158.

Cooper JA, White DA, Matthay RA: Drug-induced pulmonary disease. Parts I & II. *Am Rev Respir Dis* 1986; 133:321-340 and 133:488-505.

Fraser RG, Pare JAP: *Diagnosis of Diseases of the Chest*, ed 2. Philadelphia, WB Saunders, 1979, vol-III.

Kangarloo H, Beachley MC, Ghahremani GG: The radiographic spectrum of pulmonary complications in burn victims. *AJR* 1977; 128:441-445.

Libshitz HI: *Radiation Changes in the Lung: Conventional Studies in CT*. American Roentgen Ray Society Categorical Course Syllabus, 1986, pp 111, 119.

Meyer JE: Thoracic effects of therapeutic irradiation for breast carcinoma. *AJR* 1978; 130:877-885.

Paredes H: Radiologic evaluation of patients with chest trauma. *Med Clin North Am* 1975; 59:37-64.

Roswit B, White DC: Severe radiation injuries of the lung. *AJR* 1977; 129:127-136.

Sostman HD, Putman CE, Gamsu G: Diagnosis of chemotherapy lung. *AJR* 1981; 136:33-40.

Stewart JR, Fajardo LF: Radiation-induced heart disease: An update. *Prog Cardiovas Dis* 1984; 3:173-194.

Teixidor HS, Rubin E, Novick GS, et al: Smoke inhalation, radiologic manifestations. *Radiology* 1983; 149:383-387.

12

Chronic Infiltrative Lung Disease

Howard Mann, M.D.

KEY CONCEPTS

1. Diffuse infiltration may produce small irregular and nodular shadows, and septal lines. However, the radiograph may be normal.
2. The formation of small cystic spaces may result from cellular necrosis in small nodules, and from focal air-trapping/emphysema. It may not represent diffuse interstitial fibrosis.
3. Cystic spaces in association with reduced static lung volumes is a reliable sign of irreversible parenchymal loss.
4. Pattern recognition should never be applied in isolation; correlation should be made with relevant clinical, historical, and occupational information.

This section deals with those disorders that primarily affect the interstitial compartment of the lung. This compartment consists of the axial (peribronchovascular), parenchymal (interalveolar septa), and peripheral subpleural interstitium. The descriptor "infiltration" is used in the pathologic sense, in which any substance or cell type spreads through the interstices of the lung and accumulates in greater than normal quantity. The nature and pattern of pulmonary infiltration will reflect accumulation of one or more of the following (selected common causes are cited):

1. Fluid: interstitial edema, blood;
2. Diffuse cellular infiltrate: malignant (adenocarcinoma, lymphoma) or benign (pulmonary eosinophilia, polymorphous lymphocytic infiltrate);
3. Organized cellular aggregates: granuloma, rheumatoid nodule;
4. Organic material: amyloid, collagen, lipid;
5. Inorganic material: silica, coal, asbestos.

The inflammatory process that accompanies these infiltrative disorders may result in diffuse interstitial fibrosis. The extent of fibrosis and cystic disease due to progressive destruction of alveolar septa will determine the magnitude of clinical disability and the patient's prognosis.

The following discussion includes an overview of the radiography of diffuse infiltrative disease, a description of selected infiltrative disorders, and a diagnostic approach to interstitial infiltration and fibrosis.

RADIOGRAPHY OF DIFFUSE INFILTRATIVE PULMONARY DISEASE

The radiographic appearance depends on the nature, extent, and location of the infiltrative process. Infiltration of the peribronchovascular connective tissue sheaths (axial interstitium) will result in apparent bronchial wall thickening. The peribronchial cuffs of fluid in hydrostatic pulmonary edema are a prime example. However, tumor cell infiltration may result in an identical appearance (e.g., Hodgkin's lymphoma extending into the lung from the mediastinum; diffuse, metastatic carinomatosis).

Involvement of the subpleural interstitium is recognized directly as apparent thickening of the interlobar fissures or indirectly as thickened septal lines, as there is continuity between these two compartments. Extensive fibrosis affecting the subpleural interstitium may result in a thickened visceral pleural membrane;

this occurs in severe cases of interstitial fibrosis resulting from exposure to asbestos.

Cellular infiltration and deposition of collagen in alveolar septa will result in small irregular and small nodular shadows. This has been termed a "reticulonodular pattern." Subsequent destruction of alveolar septa will eventually result in cystic areas of variable sizes. Small cystic areas, 5 to 10 mm in diameter, may represent the radiographic correlate of pathologic "honeycombing." Small nodular shadows may also reflect the presence of noncaseating granulomas, the fibrotic nodules related to deposition of coal and silica dust, and foreign-body granulomas associated with chronic aspiration of food particles or lipid material (exogenous lipoid pneumonia).

Diffuse interstitial fibrosis will result in decreased static lung volumes (total lung capacity, vital capacity, residual volume). Diminishing lung volumes is a useful radiographic sign of progressive fibrosis.

When there is marked infiltration and expansion of the parenchymal interstitium, the differentiation between interstitial and primary air-space (alveolar) disease may be impossible. The resultant parenchymal opacities may be inhomogeneous, confluent, and poorly marginated; air bronchograms may be seen. Such opacities may be seen, for example, in sarcoidosis (interstitial granulomas) and in the reparative stage of diffuse alveolar damage (interstitial fibrosis). In diseases such as desquamative interstitial pneumonia, in which there is concurrent involvement of the interstitium (fibrosis) and alveoli (desquamated cells), similar radiographic findings may be present.

The chest radiograph may be normal in the presence of diffuse lung infiltration. Patients may present with dyspnea, rales, reduced vital capacity, and reduction in the single-breath diffusing capacity for carbon monoxide. The most common diagnoses found on open lung biopsy are sarcoidosis, desquamative interstitial pneumonia, hypersensitivity pneumonitis, and inorganic pneumoconiosis such as asbestosis. This reflects the fact that the accumulation of cells/fibrous tissue in a diffuse, nonlocalized manner may not result in discernible radiographic shadows.

SPECIFIC INFILTRATIVE DISORDERS

Usual Interstitial Pneumonia

There are many synonyms for usual interstitial pneumonia (UIP), each reflecting the accumulation of fibrous tissue in the parenchymal interstitium. The most commonly used are "idiopathic pulmonary fibrosis" and "fibrosing alveolitis." However, UIP is not a specific disease entity and may be seen in many diverse disorders such as the collagen vascular diseases, pneumoconioses, reactions to drugs, and in a heritable, familial form. The idiopathic form represents a diagnosis of exclusion.

In disorders associated with UIP, parenchymal fibrosis is often progressive and is accompanied by alveolar septal destruction (alveolar simplification) and bronchiolectasis. Cystic change becomes apparent, and small cystic spaces 5 to 10 mm in diameter may represent pathologic "honeycombing."

Pathogenetically, fibrosis is probably the end-result of an episode or repeated episodes of acute alveolitis/diffuse alveolar damage. The cells intimately associated with the acute event and ensuing fibrosis are the macrophage, neutrophil, and fibroblast. Bronchoalveolar lavage performed during the time of "active" alveolitis usually reveals abnormally high numbers of neutrophils in the aspirated fluid. Importantly, the alveolitis stage is usually subclinical, and patients typically present with progressive dyspnea as a manifestation of diffuse fibrosis.

Pathologic examination of the lung typically reveals a mixture of "early" and "late" lesions, with random distribution of lesions within the lung. Early lesions consist of widening of the alveolar septa with a mixed cellular infiltrate of mononuclear cells, active regeneration of alveolar epithelium, and patchy alveolar exudates. Late lesions show destruction of alveolar septa and interstitial fibrosis.

Radiography

Interstitial fibrosis manifests as small, irregular shadows throughout the lungs. Because attenuation of x-ray photons is relatively greatest in the lower lungs where there is more lung tissue, these small shadows are more apparent in the lung bases. Small cystic spaces may be seen, but these are never associated with fluid levels. Static lung volumes decrease with progressive fibrosis. Fibrosis is uncommonly associated with a complicating pneumothorax. Finally, dilatation of the pulmonary arteries may be seen as a manifestation of pulmonary hypertension/cor pulmonale.

Desquamative Interstitial Pneumonia

This idiopathic condition is diagnosed on lung biopsy. Some investigators believe it is an early form of interstitial fibrosis, with progression from a pattern of desquamative interstitial pneumonia (DIP) to UIP as progressive fibrosis ensues.

Pathologically, there is a prominent accumulation of cells in the alveolar spaces, primarily macrophages. Similar intra-alveolar accumulation of macrophages may be seen at the margins of the stellate nodules of primary pulmonary histiocytosis. Interstitial fibrosis and septal destruction are not a feature.

The importance of diagnosing this disorder relates to a well-documented response to steroid therapy in many patients.

Radiography

Small, irregular shadows predominate at the lung bases. Thus, this condition may be indistinguishable from UIP. However, DIP should be suspected whenever ill-defined, nonsegmental, "ground-glass" opacities are present. Small cystic spaces (5 to 10 mm) are not usually seen.

Pulmonary Lymphoid Hyperplasia

This descriptive term encompasses a spectrum of disorders associated with a polymorphous accumulation of lymphocytes and plasma cells in the lung.

Diffuse lymphoid hyperplasia (lymphocytic interstitial pneumonitis, or LIP) may be seen in association with a variety of disorders such as Sjögren's syndrome, chronic active hepatitis, pernicious anemia, rheumatoid arthritis, and, importantly, the acquired immunodeficiency syndrome (AIDS). It is often accompanied by a dysgammaglobulinemia, frequently a polyclonal gammopathy.

The interstitial lymphoid infiltrate is localized to the parenchymal, subpleural and peribronchovascular interstitium. Cytologically, the infiltrating cells are small, noncleaved lymphocytes and plasma cells. The development of enlarged hilar and/or mediastinal lymph nodes may herald the development of a malignant lymphoma, especially in Sjögren's syndrome. Fibrosis may complicate long-standing LIP, resulting in cystic change and reduced lung volumes.

Nodular lymphoid hyperplasia (pseudolymphoma) is a localized form of LIP. It is usually an isolated finding and presents as a round mass in a lung. It may compress adjacent vessels and airways, but true infiltration of these structures does not occur. Regional lymph node enlargement should not be present.

Follicular hyperplasia of submucosal, bronchus-associated lymphoid tissue may also be included in the spectrum of pulmonary lymphoid hyperplasia. It may be a pathologic finding in the lungs of patients with AIDS.

Localized, nodular lymphocytic infiltrates associated with necrosis of normal tissue may be found in the lung in angiocentric T-cell lymphoma. The nodular masses may simulate those of Wegener's granulomatosis. The lymphocytic aggregates are angiocentric/angiodestructive, a finding not present in the benign pulmonary hyperplasias.

Radiography

LIP presents as diffuse, small, irregular and nodular shadows. In severe cases, coalescence of nodules may form ill-defined, nonsegmental shadows, simulating alveolar consolidation. The occurrence of diffuse fibrosis will be associated with diminution of lung volumes and the appearance of cystic change.

Pseudolymphoma appears as a localized mass, frequently with air bronchograms. The latter indicate the bronchocentric nature of the lymphocytic infiltrate. The margin of the mass is usually not sharply defined. Associated regional lymph node enlargement should suggest the presence of a malignant lymphoma.

Computed tomography (CT) of the lungs may be diagnostically useful when pulmonary lymphoid hyperplasia is suspected. As the lymphocytic infiltrates frequently involve the peribronchovascular and septal interstitium, thickened bronchovascular bundles and septal lines/nodules may be seen, especially on high-resolution images. This appearance will also suggest a potentially high yield from transbronchoscopic biopsy. CT scanning will also help determine the presence or absence of regional lymph node enlargement in equivocal cases.

Sarcoidosis

This disorder of unknown cause is characterized by the formation of noncaseating granulomas in multiple organs, including the lung and thoracic lymph nodes. The pathogenesis of granulomatous diseases involves an amplified immune response to an inciting agent, which may or may not be known. The immune response involves primarily pulmonary macrophages and T-lymphocytes, which release various soluble cytokines that mediate the immune reaction. The end-result is the formation of an active granuloma, which consists of a central follicle of macrophages, epithelioid, and multinucleated giant cells, surrounded by a perimeter of lymphocytes, monocytes, and fibroblasts. Activated fibroblasts are responsible for the associated fibrosis.

There is a poor correlation between the appearance of the chest radiograph and pulmonary function tests, with the exception of the patient with severe, end-stage pulmonary fibrosis.

Pulmonary sarcoidosis is usually diagnosed by performing transbronchoscopic biopsy, even in patients with radiographically normal lungs. Steroid treatment may be useful in selected patients, particularly those with hypercalcemia.

Radiography

Parenchymal and/or nodal disease may be present on the chest radiograph. Parenchymal disease usually takes the form of small irregular and nodular shadows. Predominant upper lobe involvement is common. Rarely, a miliary pattern of 1- to 2-mm nodules throughout both lungs may be seen. In patients with severe fibrosis, upper lobe cystic disease may develop. At this time, lung volumes are typically very low. An associated complication is the formation of a mycetoma in a parenchymal cavity, which in turn may cause severe pulmonary hemorrhage.

Bilateral hilar lymph node enlargement is a classic finding in sarcoidosis. Mediastinal lymph nodes, particularly the right paratracheal nodes, may be enlarged. Rarely, anterior and/or posterior mediastinal lymph nodes may be enlarged. Marked involvement of the mediastinum by sarcoid granulomas may lead to compression/narrowing of structures such as pulmonary veins. Such involvement is best evaluated with CT or magnetic resonance imaging.

Sarcoid granulomas within the bronchial submucosa may cause an intrinsic bronchial stenosis. Proximal atelectasis may occur, and will not resolve on antibiotic therapy for presumed pneumonia.

Sarcoidal involvement of the trachea may result in diffuse tracheal narrowing.

The appearance of the chest radiograph at initial presentation may be used to assign patients to one of three groups. This division is based on observed differences in the rate of spontaneous resolution or improvement of the disease, as outlined in Table 12–1.

The resolution rate is higher if patients present with acute symptoms such as fever, malaise, and/or erythema nodosum. In addition, lack of radiographic resolution does not exclude the possibility of symptomatic improvement in an individual patient.

Primary Pulmonary Histiocytosis

This disease, previously called pulmonary eosinophilic granuloma, is characterized by the accumulation of atypical histiocytes in the form of parenchymal nodules. Traditionally, this disorder has been grouped with Letterer-Siwe and Hand-Schüller-Christian disease under the encompassing term "histiocytosis X." These latter two diseases are multisystem disorders that typically affect children, with a high frequency of osseous involvement. In contrast, pulmonary histiocytosis affects adults and remains confined to the lung in the vast majority of patients.

On pathologic examination, the lesions do not consist of true granulomas, and the presence of eosinophils is inconstant. The atypical histiocytes have been characterized as Langerhans' cells, derived from the bone marrow. These cells have large, convoluted nuclei, contain specific pentolaminar inclusions on electron microscopy (X-bodies) and stain positively for S-100 protein in the cytoplasm. Thus, this disease should properly be termed "Langerhans' cell histiocytosis." The parenchymal nodules are cellular, with occasional central necrosis/cavitation.

Chronic disease may be associated with diffuse expansion of alveolar septa and cystic disease. Cystic disease may reflect necrosis of cellular nodules rather than pathologic "honeycombing." Nodular involvement of the pleura may be complicated by recurrent pneumothoraces.

Radiography
Small nodular and irregular shadows are seen, pre-

TABLE 12–1.
Radiographic Presentation and Resolution Rates in Sarcoidosis

Group	Radiograph	Resolution Rate (%)
I	Hilar adenopathy alone	65–80
II	Nodal and parenchymal disease	49–68
III	Parenchymal disease alone	20–68

dominantly in the upper lung zones. The margins of the nodules are usually ill-defined, corresponding to their stellate appearance on microscopic examination. Typically, there is sparing of the costophrenic angles. These shadows may increase in size and number as the disease progresses. In the chronic form, small cystic spaces may be evident. These cystic spaces may "disappear" as the disease spontaneously subsides, serving to differentiate this disease from other causes of diffuse, interstitial fibrosis. Unlike other chronic infiltrative diseases associated with diffuse interstitial fibrosis, lung volumes are maintained, also serving as a useful differentiating feature. A pneumothorax may be present. Lymph node enlargement and pleural thickening are not a feature.

Pulmonary Lymphangiomyomatosis

This rare disorder typically affects young women, 20 to 40 years of age, who present with progressively worsening dyspnea. The disease may occur in a primary form or in association with tuberous sclerosis. Common complications are recurrent pneumothoraces and chylous effusions.

Pathologic examination of the lung reveals characteristic proliferation of smooth muscle in peribronchial, perivascular, and perilymphatic locations. Cystic change may be seen, probably resulting from focal air-trapping caused by bronchiolar occlusion. While fibrous tissue may be increased in some patients, diffuse interstitial fibrosis is not a feature of this disease.

Radiography

Lung volumes are normal or increased. Small, irregular shadows with cystic change is the characteristic appearance. Pleural fluid may represent a chylothorax. A pneumothorax may be present. While thoracic lymph nodes may contain abnormal amounts of smooth muscle, lymph node enlargement is not a radiographic finding.

Rheumatoid Arthritis

Infiltrative disease of the lung is a common occurrence in rheumatoid arthritis. The term "rheumatoid lung disease" encompasses several different causes and patterns of lung infiltration, which may present with similar radiographic findings. In addition, there is poor correlation between histologic/radiographic findings and the results of pulmonary function tests. However, the nature of the infiltrate determines the means of therapy and the prognosis.

Lung biopsies in rheumatoid arthritis may reveal one or more of the following histologic features:

1. Rheumatoid nodules (necrobiotic nodules). These nodules are composed of a central area of fibrinoid necrosis surrounded by pallisaded histiocytes and occasional giant cells. The histologic appearance is the same for nodules in extrapulmonary sites. Rheumatoid nodules are usually found adjacent to a pleural surface and in interlobular septa.

2. Usual interstitial pneumonia. In rheumatoid arthritis UIP is characterized by the occurrence of both "early" and "late" lesions, as described earlier. Thus, it is indistinguishable from other causes of diffuse, interstitial fibrosis.

3. Bronchiolitis obliterans, organizing pneumonia. Unlike the histologic picture of UIP, in bronchiolitis obliterans, organizing pneumonia (BOOP) there are plugs of young granulation tissue in the distal bronchiolar lumens, alveolar ducts, and alveoli. Small foci of obstructive pneumonia with accumulation of cholesterol-laden macrophages may be seen proximal to occluded bronchioles.

4. Lymphoid hyperplasia and cellular interstitial pneumonia. Interstitial lymphoid follicles are present along lymphatic pathways adjacent to bronchovascular bundles and in interlobular septa. When a prominent interstitial infiltration of lymphocytes and plasma cells is seen, a cellular interstitial pneumonia is also present.

Patients with UIP have the worst prognosis. BOOP may resolve with steroid therapy. Patients with rheumatoid nodules only have an excellent prognosis.

Secondary Causes of Infiltrative Disease in Rheumatoid Arthritis.— Secondary causes include pulmonary reactions to drugs (methotrexate, gold, and penicillamine) and secondary pulmonary amyloidosis.

Radiography

Rheumatoid nodules are typically well marginated and peripherally located. Cavitation may be seen as a result of central necrosis. Rarely, rheumatoid nodules may appear before the onset of clinical arthritis.

UIP, lymphoid hyperplasia, and cellular interstitial pneumonia may present as diffuse, small, irregular shadows. Progressive fibrosis in UIP manifests as diminishing lung volumes.

The appearance of BOOP is usually one of bilateral, nonsegmental, localized consolidation. The appearance has been described as that of "ground glass," and is thus quite different from that of UIP.

Scleroderma (Progressive Systemic Sclerosis)

Scleroderma and the CREST syndrome (*c*alcinosis, *R*aynaud's phenomenon, *e*sophageal disease, *s*clerodactyly, *t*elangiectasia) are closely related disorders. Pulmonary involvement is common, but radiographs are frequently normal. As with extrathoracic organ involvement, deposition of fibrous tissue is the predominant histologic finding. An additional feature of pulmonary disease, particularly in the CREST syndrome, is an occlusive vascular process that may lead to severe pulmonary hypertension.

Radiography

Interstitial fibrosis produces small irregular and linear shadows, particularly in the lower lungs. Progressive fibrosis leads to cystic change and diminishing lung volumes. Signs of pulmonary hypertension are dilatation of the main and central elastic pulmonary arteries. If severe esophageal dysmotility or an esophageal stricture is present, a dilated esophagus may be evident. The dilated esophagus may contain ingested food particles and/or a fluid level. Poorly marginated, localized opacities in the lower lobes may represent consolidation/atelectasis from episodes of aspiration pneumonia. If there is concurrent involvement of the lower gastrointestinal tract, dilated bowel loops will be seen below variably elevated hemidiaphragms.

Systemic Lupus Erythematosis

True infiltrative lung disease is not a feature of systemic lupus erythematosus (SLE). Basal interstitial fibrosis has been described, but its relationship to SLE is uncertain. Thoracic manifestations generally include one or more of the following:

1. Pleuritis and pericarditis: pleural/pericardial effusions;
2. Pulmonary capillaritis: consolidation due to hemorrhage;
3. Diffuse alveolar damage: diffuse, bilateral consolidation;
4. Diaphragmatic dysfunction: decreased lung volumes;
5. Lupus cardiomyopathy: signs of left ventricular failure.

Pulmonary Hemosiderosis

Repeated episodes of pulmonary hemorrhage may result in variable degrees of interstitial fibrosis as hemosiderin and hemosiderin-containing macrophages accumulate in the interstitium. Established causes include mitral stenosis, exposure to chemicals (trimellitic anhydride), Goodpasture's syndrome, and primary pulmonary hemosiderosis. The latter is a diagnosis of exclusion.

Radiography

Acute pulmonary hemorrhage produces consolidation, which resolves over 24 to 72 hours. Repeated episodes of hemorrhage will result in small nodular and irregular shadows, particularly in the lower lung zones. In chronic mitral stenosis, calcification and ossification of these small nodules may occur, and this may be apparent on conventional radiographs.

Pulmonary Eosinophilia

Infiltration of the pulmonary interstitium with eosinophils has been described in many diverse disorders (Table 12-2). The pathogenesis frequently involves a hypersensitivity immune response to a specific antigen, which may or may not be known. Pulmonary infiltrates with eosinophilia (PIE) refers to the presence of parenchymal opacities with peripheral eosinophilia. It is a descriptive term, and lung biopsy is rarely necessary for diagnosis and patient management.

Radiography

Eosinophilic interstitial infiltration may not be evident on a chest radiograph in the absence of associated alveolar exudate. In chronic eosinophilic pneumonia, bilateral consolidation is often present, with a predilection for peripheral lung zone involvement (reverse pulmonary edema pattern). With the other causes listed in Table 12-2, nonspecific patterns of pulmonary opacification may be seen.

Pulmonary Amyloidosis

Amyloidosis represents the extracellular deposition of fibrils derived from the light chains of monoclonal immunoglobulin. The protein is termed AL (immunoglobulin-derived amyloid). Uncommonly, the lung may be infiltrated with amyloid in the presence of chronic extrapulmonary inflammation/infection such as rheumatoid arthritis and osteomyelitis. In this situation, the amyloid consists of AA protein (a portion of the nonimmunoglobulin serum precursor SAA). The patho-

Chronic Infiltrative Lung Disease

TABLE 12-2.
Range of Disorders Found in PIE

Disorder	Key Clinical Features
Chronic eosinophilic pneumonia	Severe symptoms, steroid responsive/dependent
Löffler's syndrome	Mild symptoms, self limited
Chronic asthma	Allergic bronchopulmonary aspergillosis, Churg-Strauss phenomenon
Parasitic infection	Larval migration (e.g., *Ascaris*, *Strongyloides*)
Hypersensitivity reaction	Drugs (e.g., nitrofurantoin)
Hypereosinophilic syndrome	Myocardial infiltration. Congestive heart failure

logic diagnosis requires Congo red staining of tissue and the observation of green birefringence under the polarizing microscope.

Pulmonary parenchymal involvement generally takes two forms: localized and diffuse. Pulmonary involvement as part of systemic amyloidosis is common, but is usually of no clinical significance. Cardiac infiltration with resultant congestive heart failure is usually responsible for symptoms such as dyspnea. The localized form of pulmonary amyloidosis has a good prognosis. If suspected, the diagnosis may be made by percutaneous needle or transbronchial biopsy, obviating need for a thoracotomy.

Radiography

Diffuse infiltration of the parenchymal interstitium may be associated with a normal chest radiograph or the presence of diffuse, small irregular and nodular shadows. In the systemic form of the disease, signs of left ventricular failure may predominate.

Localized lung involvement typically presents with nodular opacities of variable size. These may slowly increase in size with observation. The nodules are often mistaken for primary bronchogenic carcinoma.

DIAGNOSTIC APPROACH TO DIFFUSE INFILTRATIVE DISEASE AND INTERSTITIAL FIBROSIS

Radiologists are frequently presented with radiographs that show diffuse parenchymal shadowing indicative of infiltrative disease and/or interstitial fibrosis. In this situation, pattern recognition may serve to limit the number of possible diagnoses. However, this approach should not be applied in isolation; relevant historical, occupational, and clinical information should always be obtained. If available, previous radiographs should be obtained for comparison.

PATTERN RECOGNITION AND DESCRIPTION OF RADIOGRAPHIC SHADOWS

Pattern recognition involves the appreciation of abnormal nonvascular, nonbronchial shadows in the lungs. When the abnormal shadows are subtle (low profusion), properly exposed radiographs are essential; overexposed radiographs will render small irregular and nodular shadows invisible. Instead of using histologic terms such as "interstitial" to describe abnormal shadows, descriptive terminology should be employed whenever a discernible pattern or combination of patterns is present. The following terms should be used:

- Small irregular shadows;
- Small nodular shadows (up to 10 mm in diameter);
- Miliary nodules (1 to 2 mm in diameter);
- Septal (Kerley) lines; and/or
- Cystic change.

It should be noted that, with the exception of cystic change, all these shadows may be seen in acute conditions such as interstitial edema and viral pneumonia, and are not diagnostic of chronic infiltration/fibrosis. The presence of cystic spaces in association with diminished lung volumes is a reliable indication of irreversible parenchymal loss.

Ring shadows may represent thickened bronchial walls and/or bronchiectasis, and should not be confused with the cystic spaces associated with septal destruction and alveolar simplification. Fibrosis may be associated with traction bronchiectasis, but fluid levels are never seen. In difficult cases, CT scanning of the lungs will serve to differentiate between these two causes of cystic disease. The cystic spaces of cystic bronchiectasis will be seen to be associated with pulmonary artery branches, giving rise to a signet-ring appearance.

SELECTED REFERENCES

Citro LA, Gordon ME, Miller WT: Eosinophilic lung disease. *AJR* 1973; 117:787.

Corrin B, Liebow AA, Friedman PJ: Pulmonary lymphangiomyomatosis. *Am J Pathol* 1975; 79:348.

Crystal RG, Bitterman PB, Rennard SI, et al: Interstitial lung diseases of unknown cause. *N Engl J Med* 1984; 310:154.

Crystal RG, Fulmer JD, Roberts WC, et al: Idiopathic pulmonary fibrosis. *Ann Intern Med* 1976; 85:769.

Epler GR, McCloud TC, Gaensler EA, et al: Normal chest roentgenograms in chronic diffuse infiltrative lung disease. *N Engl J Med* 1978; 298:934.

Felson B: A new look at pattern recognition of diffuse pulmonary disease. *AJR* 1979; 133:183.

Friedman PJ, Liebow AA, Sokoloff J: Eosinophilic granuloma of lung: Clinical aspects of primary pulmonary histiocytosis in the adult. *Medicine (Baltimore)* 1981; 60:385.

Genereux GP: Radiologic assessment of diffuse lung disease, in Taveras JM, Ferrucci JT (eds): *Radiology. Diagnosis-Imaging-Intervention*. Philadelphia, JB Lippincott Co, 1986, vol 1.

Gross BH, Felson B, Birnberg FA: The respiratory tract in amyloidosis and the plasma cell dyscrasias. *Semin Roentgenol* 1986; 21:113.

Kradin RL, Mark EJ: Benign lymphoid disorders of the lung, with a theory regarding their development. *Hum Pathol* 1983; 14:857.

Pines A, Kaplinsky N, Olchovsky D, et al: Pleuropulmonary manifestations of SLE: Clinical features of its subgroups. *Chest* 1985; 88:129.

Rockoff SD, Rohatgi PK: Unusual manifestations in thoracic sarcoidosis. *AJR* 1985; 144:513.

Scott PP, Scott WW, Siegelman SS: Amyloidosis: An overview. *Semin Roentgenol* 1986; 21:103.

Shiel WC, Prete PE: Pleuropulmonary manifestations of rheumatoid arthritis. *Semin Arthritis Rheum* 1984; 13:235.

Thomas PD, Hunninghake GW: Current concepts of the pathogenesis of sarcoidosis. *Am Rev Respir Dis* 1987; 135:747.

Valdivia E, Hensley G, Wu J, et al: Morphology and pathogenesis of desquamative interstitial pneumonitis. *Thorax* 1977; 32:7.

Yousem SA, Colby TV, Carrington CB: Lung biopsy in rheumatoid arthritis. *Am Rev Respir Dis* 1985; 131:770.

13 | Chest Radiography in the Intensive Care Unit

Howard Mann, M.D.

KEY CONCEPTS

1. Daily conferences establishing communication between radiologist and physicians in the intensive care unit are essential.
2. The location of tubes, drains, and catheters should be evaluated. Barotrauma should be excluded.
3. The assessment of diffuse disease should take into account mode of ventilation and lung volumes. Radiographic density is dependent on the relative amounts of lung water, tissue, and air.
4. Serial assessment of radiographs is essential when determining intravascular fluid status and evaluating extravascular lung water.
5. Radiographs are reliable when extravascular lung water is identified. Intravascular pressure measurements are not a standard against which clinical and radiographic findings should be judged.

This chapter is intended to provide the radiologist and critical care physician with a systematic approach to the interpretation of chest radiographs obtained in intensive care units (ICUs). The following discussion will also focus on pertinent technical aspects of bedside radiography that affect image interpretation.

MOBILE RADIOGRAPHY

Chest radiographs obtained with mobile radiographic units differ from conventional radiographs in several important respects, primarily in exposure times, patient positioning, and exposure latitude, radiographic contrast, and kilovolt (peak) [kV(p)].

Exposure Times

Exposure times are relatively long in mobile units compared with radiographs obtained with conventional three-phase generators. This, coupled with the inability of critically ill patients to suspend respiration, often results in loss of edge detail, with the unsharpness due to patient motion. Vascular margins may appear indistinct, and this should not be misinterpreted as interstitial edema, particularly in the absence of other signs such as peribronchial cuffs and septal lines.

Patient Positioning

Chest radiographs in the ICU frequently have to be taken with the patient supine or semierect. There is often associated caudal or cranial beam angulation relative to the film cassette, resulting in apparent diaphragmatic elevation and effacement of the hemidiaphragmatic contour. The latter in particular may result in the erroneous diagnosis of lower lobe disease. When this result is anticipated, a well-centered radiograph taken with the patient supine has much greater diagnostic efficacy. A standard source-to-image receptor distance should be established to facilitate comparison of cardiac and vascular dimensions with their appearance in previous and succeeding radiographs.

Exposure Latitude, Radiographic Contrast, and Kilovolt (Peak)

Bedside radiographs are obtained at a lower kV(p) setting [80 to 90 kV(p)] than is used in conventional radiographs [120 to 140 kV(p)]. Exposure latitude (the range of exposures that will result in an appropriate optical density) is less with lower kV(p) levels. This fact, coupled with the need for manual exposures, accounts for the frequent daily variation in optical density. With lower kilovoltage settings, more radiation passes through the lungs than through the mediastinum. This large dynamic range of information may exceed the ability of conventional film-screen combinations to record and display with sufficient radiographic contrast. Exposure often occurs near the toe of the H & D curve, resulting in inadequate display of mediastinal and retrocardiac structures (Fig 13–1). Inability to visualize the descending aorta and retrocardiac parenchymal structures, for example, may reflect this technical limitation of bedside radiography rather than a true disease condition.

AN APPROACH TO RADIOGRAPHIC INTERPRETATION

An orderly approach to the ICU radiograph should include an assessment of the following features:

- Mode of respiration/ventilation and lung volumes;
- Placement of intravascular catheters, tubes, and drains;
- Barotrauma;
- Extravascular and intravascular fluid status; and
- Progression/regression of known cardiopulmonary disease.

Mode of Respiration/Ventilation and Lung Volumes

Patients may be breathing spontaneously or may be mechanically ventilated. Positive pressure ventilation is commonly applied utilizing IPPV (intermittent positive pressure ventilation), CPAP (continuous positive airway pressure), or PEEP (positive end-expiratory pressure). Whenever possible, radiographs of mechan-

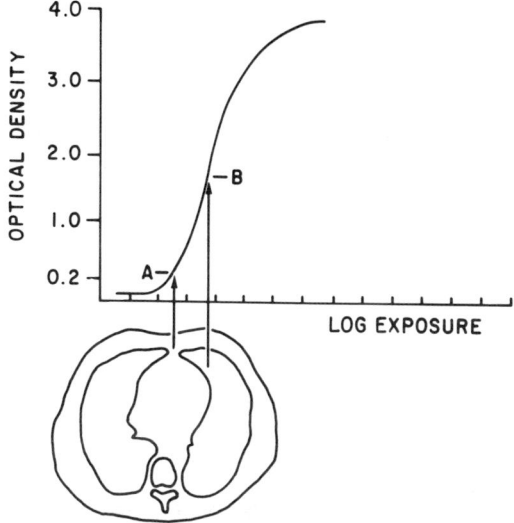

FIG 13–1.
Radiographic exposure difference between lung and mediastinum. (On bedside radiographs, the value for the mediastinum may fall on the toe of the H & D curve.) *A*, optical density = 0.3 (underexposed); *B*, optical density = 1.7 (adequately exposed).

ically ventilated patients should be exposed at the end of the inspiratory phase of the ventilatory cycle, thus facilitating comparison with earlier and subsequent radiographs.

In patients with extensive air-space consolidation, varying lung volumes will change the apparent extent and distribution of alveolar fluid. Perceived optical density reflects the relative amounts of fluid and air in the lung. Application of positive airway pressure with a

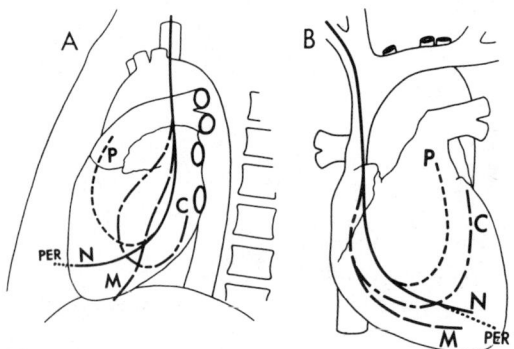

FIG 13–2.
Pacemaker lead positions in the frontal and lateral projections. (*N* = right ventricular apex; *P* = main pulmonary artery; *M* = middle cardiac vein; *C* = coronary sinus; *Per* = perforating lead.) (From Steiner RM, Tegtmeyer CJ, Morse D, et al: The radiology of cardiac pacemakers. *RadioGraphics* 1986; 6:373-399. Reproduced by permission.)

resultant increase in lung volumes will result in "pseudoresolution" of air-space consolidation.

Increasing lung volumes with application of positive airway pressures may also lead to a decrease in the width of the vascular mediastinum. The width of the vascular pedicle (defined in Fig 4-2), which is used to assess total circulating blood volume, may decrease. This relates to the fact that the caliber of a mediastinal vessel is a reflection of transmural pressure, which will decrease when extravascular, mediastinal pressure is increased by the application of CPAP or PEEP.

Thus, the mode of ventilation and lung volumes should always be taken into account when evaluating and comparing bedside radiographs obtained in the ICU.

Chest Radiography in the ICU **215**

TABLE 13–1.
Catheters, Tubes, and Leads Seen in ICU Patients

Endotracheal tube
Tracheostomy tube
Central venous catheter
Swan-Ganz catheter
Intra-aortic balloon pump
Pacemaker leads
Thoracostomy tube
Nasogastric and enteric tubes

Placement of Intravascular Catheters, Tubes, and Drains

The position of various catheters, leads, tubes, and drains should be evaluated next. Those commonly used are listed in Table 13–1.

Endotracheal Tube

The position of the endotracheal tube should be assessed in relation to the carina. Because the tube is usually taped to the skin of the face, its position relative to the carina will change slightly with flexion and extension of the patient's neck. The following measurements from the end of the tube to the carina indicate appropriate position in the adult:

Neck neutral	5 to 7 cm
Neck flexed	3 to 5 cm
Neck extended	7 to 9 cm

The size of the endotracheal tube cuff should be assessed in relation to the coronal diameter of the trachea. Marked overinflation of the cuff relative to the coronal diameter of the trachea, particularly with distal extension of the cuff toward the end of the tube, may indicate "occult" tracheal rupture. Another sign of tracheal rupture is the appearance of mediastinal emphysema.

Tracheostomy Tube

The tracheostomy tube should be centered in the trachea without impingement of the distal end against the lateral tracheal wall.

Central Venous Catheters

Traditionally, central venous catheters are placed in a central vein distal to the last venous valve. However, many catheters are placed for infusion of cytotoxic drugs, for hemodialysis, and for hyperalimentation rather than pressure measurement. Placement in a large, high-flow vessel should be confirmed with a chest radiograph. Central catheters are most commonly directed into the superior vena cava (SVC) from a subclavian or jugular vein. After initial placement, a pneumothorax should be "ruled-out." The catheter should be directed vertically without impingement against the lateral wall of the SVC, or with abrupt angulation at the tip, which may indicate intramural perforation. The catheter tip should not be placed in the right atrium. When triple-lumen catheters are used, one should be certain that the distal side-hole, identified by a radiopaque mark on the catheter, is within the vascular lumen.

Swan-Ganz Catheter

The tip of the Swan-Ganz catheter should be in the central left or right pulmonary artery in the region of the radiographic hilus. Distal placement of the catheter should be corrected. In addition, there should be no loops of catheter in the right atrium or ventricle, which may precipitate arrythmias and permit undetected distal migration.

Intra-aortic Balloon Pump

The distal end of the intra-aortic balloon pump catheter is located by identifying the radiopaque mark at the tip. This mark should be located just distal to the origin of the left subclavian artery in the proximal descending aorta.

Cardiac Pacemaker Leads

Permanent or temporary transvenous pacemaker leads may be present. These should be intact throughout their length and should terminate in the appropriate location: the right ventricle and/or right atrium. Common locations of malpositioned leads are illustrated in Figure 13–2.

Thoracostomy Tube

The distal tip of the tube should not abut a mediastinal structure. The distal side-hole should be identified, and one should be certain this hole is within the pleural space. If the pleural tube has been inserted to drain a localized air or fluid collection, two orthogonal projections may be needed to verify appropriate placement. These views will also permit detection of tube placement in an interlobar fissure.

Nasogastric and Enteric Feeding Tubes

Radiographs should be obtained following insertion of feeding tubes to verify appropriate placement. Feeding tubes, in particular, may inadvertently be passed into the tracheobronchial tree. Placement of the distal side-hole of the nasogastric tube through the gastroesophageal junction into the stomach should be verified.

Barotrauma

Pneumothorax, pneumomediastinum, and interstitial emphysema are manifestations of barotrauma that should be evaluated on ICU radiographs. This applies particularly to the patient being ventilated with positive airway pressures and resultant high mean airway pressure.

Radiography

A pneumothorax may be very difficult to appreciate when the radiograph is obtained with the patient supine. It may manifest as increased lucency at the base of a hemithorax about the heart (anteromedial pneumothorax) and a deep, sharp lateral costophrenic angle ("deep sulcus" sign). Whenever the margin or outline of a mediastinal structure appears unusually sharp, a pneumothorax should be suspected. If uncertainty exists, the possibility of a pneumothorax may be further evaluated with additional decubitus or horizontal-beam lateral projections.

Interstitial emphysema may manifest as irregular and linear lucencies, different from the tubular, tapering appearance of air bronchograms. A perivascular lucent halo is another sign of interstitial emphysema. Finally, when sufficient air has accumulated in the subpleural interstitium, round subpleural air cysts may be seen.

Mediastinal emphysema is usually recognizable when linear, vertically oriented streaks of air collect in the superior mediastinum, and dissect cephalad through the thoracic inlet. Subcutaneous emphysema in the soft tissues of the neck and supraclavicular regions may be present. Mediastinal air may collect around the heart, and be difficult to distinguish from a medial pneumothorax. Air may extend around the base of the heart, giving rise to a "continuous diaphragm" sign. Mediastinal air may extend caudally into the abdomen as a pneumoretroperitoneum or, uncommonly, a pneumoperitoneum.

Pneumopericardium may sometimes be difficult to distinguish from pneumomediastinum. Decubitus radiographs should be obtained. Air in the pericardial space will move away from the dependent hemithorax and will accumulate around the lower border of the heart.

Extravascular and Intravascular Fluid Status

Extravascular Lung Water

This term refers primarily to the presence of interstitial and alveolar pulmonary edema. The radiographic appearance of interstitial edema has been described in the section on pulmonary edema. As previously mentioned, the presence of signs of interstitial edema (e.g., septal lines) serves to differentiate between hydrostatic and increased-permeability pulmonary edema. At present, analysis of the chest radiograph is the only convenient, practical, and noninvasive means of evaluating extravascular lung water.

Intravascular Fluid Status

The width of the vascular pedicle correlates well with total intravascular blood volume. Pulmonary blood volume increases very slightly if at all when the circulation is "overloaded" by the administration of intravenous fluids. The large systemic veins such as the SVC act as capacitance vessels: increased transmural pressure is recognized as vascular distention. Serial evaluation of the vascular pedicle is much more useful than a single observation.

Expansion of total blood volume and the resultant increased cardiac output may be accompanied by elevated pulmonary intravascular pressures. The latter will result in distended pulmonary vessels if extravascular, transpleural pressures remain constant. However, vascular distention is not synonymous with fluid overload.

The recognition of fluid overload depends on an integration of clinical and radiographic findings. Physical examination (peripheral edema), fluid intake/fluid output data, daily weights, and urinalysis should be correlated with radiographic findings.

Hemodynamic data derived from the use of pulmonary artery occlusion catheters is frequently compared with findings on the chest radiograph. In left ventricular failure, there is an expected correlation between increasing pulmonary occlusion pressure and the development of interstitial and alveolar edema. However, there are many technical and interpretive pitfalls relating to the use of Swan-Ganz catheters, and intravascular pressure measurements should not be used as a standard against which clinical and radiographic findings should be judged.

Progression/Regression of Known Cardiopulmonary Disease

After all the features described above have been evaluated, attention should finally be directed toward the specific abnormality or abnormalities known to be present. These may include consolidation due to pneumonia, obstructive volume loss, and pleural effusions.

To obtain the greatest diagnostic yield from ICU radiographs, the following recommendations are made:

1. Daily conferences between the radiologist and the ICU team should be standard practice. This will enable meaningful integration of clinical and radiographic information.
2. Interpretation of a current radiograph should always be made in relation to previously obtained radiographs. Serial assessment of parameters such as soft tissue edema and vascular pedicle width is thus facilitated.

SELECTED REFERENCES

Carter AR, Sostman HD, Curtis AM, et al: Thoracic alterations after cardiac surgery. *AJR* 1983; 140:475.

Gates LM, Matthay MA: Central intravascular pressure measurements: When should we believe them? *J Thorac Imag* 1986; 1:52.

Goodman LR: Postoperative chest radiograph: Alterations after abdominal surgery. *AJR* 1980; 134:533.

Goodman LR: Postoperative chest radiograph: Alterations after major intrathoracic surgery. *AJR* 1980; 134:803.

Greene R: Adult respiratory distress syndrome: Acute alveolar damage. *Radiology* 1987; 163:57.

Maunder RJ, Pierson DJ, Hudson LD: Subcutaneous and mediastinal emphysema. *Arch Intern Med* 1984; 144:1447.

Mc Cloud TC, Barash PG, Ravin CE: PEEP: Radiographic features and associated complications. *AJR* 1977; 129:209.

Milne ENC: A physiologic approach to reading critical care unit films. *J Thorac Imag* 1986; 1:60.

Ovenfors C: Iatrogenic trauma to the thorax. *J Thorac Imag* 1987; 2:18.

Steiner RM, Tegtmeyer CJ, Morse D, et al: The radiology of cardiac pacemakers. *RadioGraphics* 1986; 6:373.

Tocino IM: Pneumothorax in the supine patient: Radiographic anatomy. *RadioGraphics* 1985; 5:557.

Index

A

Acinetobacter pneumonia, 29
  radiography of, 29
Actinomycosis, 42–43
  radiography of, 43
Adenomatoid malformation: cystic, in lung of newborn, 10
Adenovirus: causing pneumonia, 32–33
Adrenal corticosteroids, 55
Aerobic gram-negative organisms, 26–30
  pneumonias, pathogenesis of, 27
Aerosol exposure, 186–187
Allergic
  angiitis, 164–165
    radiography of, 165
  aspergillosis (*see* Aspergillosis, allergic)
  granulomatosis, 164–165
    radiography of, 165
Alveolar edema: distribution of, 102
Amyloidosis
  pulmonary, 204–206
    radiography of, 206
  tracheal narrowing due to, 124
Anaerobic bacillary pneumonia, 30–32
  pathogenesis, 30
Angiitis, allergic, 164–165
  radiography of, 165
Angiography
  to exclude shunt and Eisenmenger's physiology in pulmonary hypertension, 91
  pulmonary
    in pulmonary embolism, 114–115
    of pulmonary hypertension, 93–95
Anomalies: cystic adenomatoid, of lung in newborn, 10
Aortic laceration: traumatic, 175–176

Arteries: pulmonary, erosion, 40
Arteriopathy: plexogenic, and pulmonary hypertension, 92
Arteritis
  Takaysu's, 166
  temporal, 166
Arthritis (see Rheumatoid arthritis)
Asbestos: and bronchogenic carcinoma, 151–152
Asbestos-related
  fibrosis, interstitial, 151
    radiography of, 151
  parenchymal abnormalities, 151–154
  pleural disease, 147–151
  pleural effusion, 147–148
Asbestosis, 146–147, 151
  epidemiology, 146–147
  pathogenesis, 147
  radiography of, 151
Aspergillosis, 49–51
  allergic bronchopulmonary, 50–51, 130–132
    diagnosis, criteria for, 131
    radiography of, 51
  invasive, 50
    radiography of, 50
  mycetoma in, 49
    radiography of, 49
  semi-invasive, 50
    radiography of, 50
Aspiration
  pneumonia (see Pneumonia, aspiration)
  syndromes, 30–32
    radiography of, 31
Asthma, 129–130
  radiography of, 129–130
Atelectasis, rounded, 149–150
  radiography of, 150
Atelectatic pseudotumor, 149–150
  radiography of, 150
Atresia
  esophagus, 12–13
  tracheoesophageal, 11
Azygous vein: and pulmonary edema, 101

B

Bacterial pneumonia, 24–34
Balloon pump: intra-aortic, 216–217
Barotrauma, 217–218
  radiography in, 217–218
Berylliosis, 154–155
  radiography, 155
Blastomycosis, North American, 48–49
  radiography of, 49
Bronchi, disease, chronic, 127–138
  definitions, 127–128
  key concepts, 127
  pathophysiology, 127–128
Bronchi: tracheobronchial fracture, 174
Bronchiectasis, 132–133
  radiography of, 133
Bronchiolitis obliterans, 136–137
  radiography of, 136–137
Bronchitis, chronic, 128–129
  radiography of, 128–129
Bronchogenic carcinoma: and asbestos, 151–152
Bronchopleural fistula: complicating tuberculosis, 39
Bronchopulmonary aspergillosis (see Aspergillosis, allergic bronchopulmonary)

dysplasia in newborn, 6–7
sequestration, 11–18
Burns, 187–188

C

Cancer
chemotherapy, 55
lung
pathologic characteristics, 74–75
radiographic features, 74–75
Candidiasis, 52
radiography of, 52
Carcinoma: bronchogenic, and asbestos, 151–152
Cardiogenic edema, 103
Catheter(s)
central venous, 216
seen in ICU, 215–217
Swan-Ganz, 216
Catheterization: cardiac, to exclude shunt and Eisenmenger's physiology in pulmonary hypertension, 91
Cavitary disease: persistent, 48
Central venous catheter, 216
Chemotherapy: of cancer, 55
Chest
abnormalities due to drugs, 182–183
neoplasms (see Neoplasms of chest)
newborn (see Newborn, chest)
radiography (see Radiography, chest)
trauma, blunt, 170–177
general features, 170–171
wall
causes of respiratory distress in newborn, 21
edema of soft tissue, 102
neoplasms, 58–60
neoplasms, radiography, 60
trauma, blunt, 171–172
Churg-Strauss phenomenon, 164–165
radiography of, 165
Cilia: primary ciliary dyskinesia, 133
Circulation: persistent fetal, 8–9
Coal worker's pneumoconiosis (see Pneumoconiosis, coal worker's)
cocci: gram-positive, 24–26
Coccidioidal pneumonia, chronic progressive, 47
radiography of, 47
Coccidioidoma: pulmonary, 48
Coccidioidomycosis, 46–48
disseminated, 48
radiography of, 48
primary, 47
radiography of, 47
"Coin lesions," 72
Connective tissue disorders
pulmonary hypertension, and, 90
tracheal dilatation in, 125
Corticosteroids: adrenal, 55
Cryptococcis, 51
radiography of, 51
Cyst: traumatic lung, 173
Cystic adenomatoid malformation: of lung in newborn, 10

Cystic fibrosis, 134–135
  radiography of, 134–135
Cytomegalovirus: causing pneumonia in immunocompromised hosts, 33

D

Diabetic mother: newborn of, 9
Diaphragmatic rupture, 176–177
Drains: placement in ICU, 215–217
Drug(s)
  chest abnormalities due to, 182–183
  ingestion and pulmonary hypertension, 90
  injury, 180–185
Dysplasia: bronchopulmonary, in newborn, 6–7

E

Echocardiography: to exclude shunt and Eisenmenger's physiology in pulmonary hypertension, 91
Edema
  alveolar, distribution of, 102
  cardiogenic, 103
  chest wall soft tissue, 102
  interstitial, 99
  pulmonary, 95–103
    azygous vein and, 101
    in emphysema, 143
    heart size and, 100
    hydrostatic, radiographic differentiation, 99–102
    increased-permeability, 103
    increased-permeability, radiographic differentiation of, 99–102
    pathophysiology, 95–97
    pleural effusion and, 101
    radiography of, 97–99
    septal lines and, 101
    vascular pedicle and, 101
Eisenmenger's physiology: excluded in pulmonary hypertension, 91
Embolism, pulmonary, 105–116
  (See also Thromboembolism, pulmonary)
  angiography of, pulmonary, 114–115
  diagnosis
    clinical, 107–116
    strategy for, 115–116
  fat, 117–118
    radiography of, 118
  imaging of, 109
  with infarction, 110–111
  pathophysiology, 106–107
  radiography of, chest, 108–110
  septic, 118–119
    radiography of, 119
  tumor, 117
    radiography of, 117
  venography of, lower limb, 108
  ventilation/perfusion scanning, 111–114
  V/Q imaging interpretation in, 113
  without infarction, 110
Embryology: of newborn chest, 2–3

Emphysema, 139–144
  centriacinar, 140
  centrilobular, 140
  CT of, 143
  definition, 139–140
  irregular, 141
  key concepts, 139
  lobal, congenital, 10
  morphologic categories, 140–141
  panacinar, 140
  paraseptal, 141
  pneumonia in, 143
  pulmonary edema in, 143
  pulmonary hypertension in, 142–143
  radiography of, 141–142
    radiolucent areas with vascular attenuation, 142
Empyema: complicating tuberculosis, 39
Endobronchial tuberculosis, 40
Endotracheal tube, 215–216
Enteric feeding tube, 217
Enterobacter pneumonia, 28–29
  radiography of, 28–29
Eosinophilia, pulmonary, 204
  radiography of, 204
  range of disorders characterized by, 205
Epstein-Barr virus: causing pneumonia, 33
Escherichia coli pneumonia, 29
  radiography of, 29
Esophagus
  atresia, 12–13
  tracheoesophageal (*see* Tracheoesophageal)

F

Fat embolism, pulmonary, 117–118
  radiography of, 118
Feeding tubes, 217
Fetal circulation: persistent, 8–9
Fever: Q fever pneumonia, 37
  asbestos-related interstitial, 151
    radiography of, 151
  cystic, 134–135
    radiography of, 134–135
  interstitial, diagnostic approach to, 206
  mediastinal, idiopathic, causing tracheal narrowing, 125
Fistula
  bronchopleural, complicating tuberculosis, 39
  tracheoesophageal, 12–13
Fluid
  accumulation in lung, sequence of, 97
  status
    extravascular, 218–219
    intravascular, 218–219
Fluoroscopy: of tracheal dynamics, 126
Fracture: tracheobronchial, 174
Fungal infection
  of lung, 43–52
  tracheal narrowing due to, 121–123

G

Gases: noxious, 186–187
Granuloma, *Histoplasma*, 45–46
  radiography of, 46

allergic, 164–165
  radiography of, 165
 Wegener's
  classification, 161–164
  radiography of, 164
  tracheal narrowing due to, 123
Granulomatous fibrosing mediastinitis, 46
 radiography of, 46

H

Heart
 catheterization to exclude shunt and Eisenmenger's physiology in pulmonary hypertension, 91
 disease, progression/regression of known, 220
 failure, congestive, in newborn, 18–19
 injuries, 174–175
 output increase in pulmonary hypertension, 88
 size in pulmonary edema, 100
Hematoma: of lung, 173–174
Hemoglobinopathy: and pulmonary hypertension, 90
Hemophilus influenzae, 27
 radiography of, 27
Hemosiderosis, pulmonary, 203–204
 radiography of, 204
Hernia: diaphragmatic, congenital, 10–11
Herpes
 simplex virus in immunocompromised hosts, 34
 varicella-zoster virus causing pneumonia
  in adults, 33
  in immunocompromised hosts, 33–34
Histiocytosis, pulmonary, 198–200
 radiography of, 198–200
Histoplasma granuloma, 45–46
 radiography of, 46
Histoplasmosis, 44–46
 chronic fibrocavitary, 45
  radiography of, 45
 disseminated, 45
  radiography of, 45
 primary pulmonary, 44–45
  radiography of, 44–45
Hodgkin's disease
 classification
  Rye, 66
  staging, 69
 pathogens in, 54
Hyaline membrane disease, 4–6
Hyperinflation: of lung, 142
Hyperplasia pulmonary, lymphoid, 195–196
 radiography of, 196
Hypersensitivity
 pneumonitis (*see* Pneumonitis, hypersensitivity)
 vasculitis, 165–166
Hypertension, pulmonary, 86–95
 angiography of, pulmonary, 93–95
 arteriopathy and, plexogenic, 92
 cardiac output increase in, 88
 connective tissue disorders and, 90

CT of, 95
definition, 86–89
diagnostis approach to, 90–93
differentiation of, 94
drug ingestion and, 90
Eisenmenger's physiology excluded in, 91
in emphysema, 142–143
hemoglobinopathy and, 90
history in, 90
imaging in, 93–95
key concepts, 86–104
liver disease and, 90
luminal diameter decrease in, 88–89
morphology, 88–89
luminal vascular obstruction in, 89
metastases and, 90
MRI of, 95
physical examination in, 90
pulmonary vascular resistance increase in, 88
pulmonary veno-occlusive disease and, 92–93
pulmonary venous pressure increase in, 88
radiography of, 89–90
radionuclide studies in, 95
shunt excluded in, 91
terminology, 86–89
thromboembolism and, pulmonary, 92
ultrasound in, 95
vascular loss in, 89
vasoconstriction in, 89

I

Imaging
of pulmonary embolism, 109
ventilation/perfusion, 111–114
of pulmonary hypertension, 93–95
of thrombosis, deep vein, 109
V/Q, interpretation in pulmonary embolism, 113
Immune complex disease: and vasculitis, 167
Immunocompromised host radiography of, chest, 53–56
viral pneumonia in, 33–34
Immunosuppressed host: predominant pathogens in specific clinical situations, 53
Infarction: in pulmonary embolism, 110–111
Infection
lung (see Lung, infection)
mycobacterial, 37–42
Influenza: in adults, 32
Inhalation injuries, 186–187
Injury (see Lung, injury)
Intensive care unit, 210–221
catheters seen in, 215–217
drain placement in, 215–217
leads seen in, 215
radiography in, chest, 210–221
interpretation approach, 212–220
key concepts, 210
tubes seen in, 215–217

K

Kilovolt: in mobile radiography, 211–212
Klebsiella pneumonia, 27–28
 radiography, 28

L

Leads: seen in ICU, 215
Legionella pneumonia, 29–30
 radiography of, 30
Leukemia: pathogens in, 54
Liver disease: and pulmonary hypertension, 90
Luminal (*see* Hypertension, pulmonary, luminal)
Lung
 (*See also* Pulmonary)
 cancer (*see* Cancer, lung)
 cavitary disease, persistent, 48
 coccidioidoma, 48
 "coin lesion," 72
 contusion, 173
 cyst, traumatic, 173
 developmental abnormalities, 9–18
 disease
  chronic infiltrative (*see below*)
  mycobacteria causing, nontuberculous, 41–42
  occupational, 145–157
  occupational, key concepts, 145–146
  progression/regression of known, 220
 disease, chronic infiltrative, 190–209
  diagnostic approach to, 206
  key concepts, 190–191
  radiographic shadows in, pattern recognition and description of, 206–207
  radiography of, 191–193
  specific disorders, 193
 dysmaturity, 7
 fluid accumulation in, sequence of, 97
 hematoma, 173–174
 hyperinflation, 142
 infection, 23–57
  fungal, 43–52
  general considerations, 23–24
  key concepts, 23
 injury, 169–189
  blunt (*see* Chest, trauma, blunt)
  key concepts, 169–189
  penetrating, 169–170
  thermal, 187–188
 laceration, 173
 mass, solitary, radiographic evaluation, 72
 metastases, 79–84
  patterns, 82
  radiography of, 83–84
  sites, probable primary, 82
 neoplasms, primary, 71–79
  radiography of, 79
 parenchymal injury, 173–174
 radiographic exposure, 213
 underdevelopment, 9–10
 volumes, 212–215
 water, extravascular, 218–219
Lupus erythematosus: systemic, 203

Lymphangiectasia: pulmonary, 18
Lymphangiomyomatosis, pulmonary, 200
  radiography of, 200
Lymphoma: non-Hodgkin's, staging classification, 69

M

Magnetic resonance imaging: of pulmonary hypertension, 95
Malformation: cystic adenomatoid, of lung, in newborn, 10
Measles
  in immunocompromised hosts, 34
  radiography of, 34
  with pneumonia, 33
Mediastinitis, granulomatous fibrosing, 46
  radiography of, 46
Mediastinum
  causing neonatal respiratory distress, 19–21
  fibrosis, idiopathic, causing tracheal narrowing, 125
  masses in newborn
    anterior, 19–20
    middle, 20
    posterior, 20–21
  neoplasms, 62–71
    incidence, 63
    location, 63
    radiography of, 71
  radiographic exposure, 213
  trauma, blunt, 174–176
Mesothelioma, malignant, 150–151
  radiography of, 150–151
Mestatases

distant, TNM definitions, 81
lung (*see* Lung, metastases)
pulmonary hypertension and, 90
Mounier-Kühn syndrome: causing tracheal widening, 125
Mycetoma
  in aspergillosis, 49
  formation, 40
Mycobacteria: nontuberculous, causing lung disease, 41–42
Mycobacterial infection, 37–42
Mycobacterium
  avium-intracellulare, 42
    radiography of, 42
  fortuitum, 42
  kansasii, 41
    radiography of, 41
Mycoplasma pneumonia (*see* Pneumonia, *Mycoplasma*)
Myeloma: multiple, pathogens in, 54

N

Naosgastric feeding tube, 217
Neoplasma
  chest, 58–85
    key concepts, 58
    wall, 58–60
    wall, radiography, 60
  lung, primary, 71–79
    radiography of, 79
  mediastinum (*see* Mediastinum, neoplasms)
  pleural, 60–62
    radiography of, 61–62
  pulmonary tumor embolism, 116–117

radiography of, 117
rib, 59
Newborn
  bronchopulmonary dysplasia, 6–7
  chest, 1–22
    embryology, 2–3
    evaluation of, considerations in, 14–17
    key concepts, 1–2
  cystic adenomatoid malformation of lung in, 10
  of diabetic mother, 9
  heart failure, congestive, 18–19
  mediastinal masses in (see Mediastinum, masses in newborn)
  pneumonia, 7–8
  respiratory distress (see Respiratory, distress in newborn)
  tachypnea, transient, 6
Nocardiosis, 43
  radiography of, 43
North American blastomycosis, 48–49
  radiography of, 49
Noxious gases, 186–187

P

Pacemaker: lead positions, 214, 217
Phycomycosis, 51–52
  radiography of, 52
Pleural
  bronchopleural fistula complicating tuberculosis, 39
  effusion
    asbestos-related, 147–148
    pulmonary edema and, 101

neoplasms, 60–62
  radiography of, 61–62
plaques, 148
  radiography of, 148–149
thickening, diffuse, 149
trauma, blunt, 172–173
Plexogenic arteriopathy: and pulmonary hypertension, 92
Pneumatocele, 173
Pneumococcal pneumonia, 24–25
  radiography of, 25
coal worker's, 153–154
  pathology, 154
  radiography of, 154
inorganic dust, 146–155
Pneumocystis carinii, 52–53
  radiography in, 53
Pneumonia
  Acinetobacter, 29
    radiography of, 29
  aerobic gram-negative, pathogenesis of, 27
  anaerobic bacillary, 30–32
    pathogenesis, 30
  aspiration, 30–32
    infectious agents in, 31
    pathogenesis, 30
  atypical, 34–37
  bacterial, 24–34
  coccidioidal, chronic progressive, 47
    radiography of, 47
  cytomegalovirus, in immunocompromised hosts, 33
  in emphysema, 143
  Enterobacter, 28
    radiography of, 28–29
  Escherichia coli, 29
    radiography of, 29
  interstitial
    desquamative, 194

desquamative, radiography of, 194
usual, 193–194
usual, radiography of, 194
Klebsiella, 27–28
radiography of, 28
Legionella, 29–30
radiography of, 30
Mycoplasma, 34–35
extrapulmonary symptoms, 36
pulmonary manifestations, 35
radiography of, 35
newborn, 7–8
pneumococcal, 24–25
radiography of, 25
Proteus, 28
radiography of, 28
Pseudomonas aeruginosa, 28
radiography of, 28
Q fever, 37
radiography of, 37
Serratia marcescens, 29
radiography of, 29
staphylococcal, 25
radiography of, 25
streptococcal, 25–26
radiography of, 26
viral, 32–34
in adults, 32–33
Epstein-Barr, 33
herpes varicella-zoster, 33
herpes varicella-zoster, in immunocompromised hosts, 33
with viral disease, systemic, 33
Pneumonitis, hypersensitivity, 155–156
clinical presentation, 156
diagnosis, 156
pathogenesis, 155–156
radiography of, 156
Polyarteritis nodosa, 165
Polychondritis: relapsing, causing tracheal narrowing, 123
Primary ciliary dyskinesia, 133
Proteus pneumonia, 28
radiography of, 28
Pseudomonas aeruginosa pneumonia, 28
radiography of, 28
Pseudotumor, atelectatic, 149–150
radiography of, 150
Psittacosis, 35
radiography of, 35
Pulmonary
(*See also* Lung)
amyloidosis, 204–206
radiography, 206
angiography (*see* Angiography, pulmonary)
artery erosion, 40
bronchopulmonary (*see* Bronchopulmonary)
causes of respiratory distress, 3–18
edema (*see* Edema, pulmonary)
embolism (*see* Embolism, pulmonary)
eosinophilia, 204
radiography of, 204
range of disorders characterized by, 205
hemosiderosis, 203–204
radiography of, 204
histiocytosis, 198–200
radiography of, 198–200
hyperplasia, lymphoid, 195–196
radiography of, 196

hypertension (see Hypertension, pulmonary)
lymphangiectasia, 18
lymphangiomyomatosis, 200
  radiography of, 200
thromboembolism (see Thromboembolism, pulmonary)
tuberculosis (see Tuberculosis, pulmonary)
vascular resistance, 87
  increase in pulmonary hypertension, 88
vasculitis (see Vasculitis, pulmonary)
veno-occlusive disease and pulmonary hypertension, 92–93
venous pressure increase in pulmonary hypertension, 88
Pump: intra-aortic balloon, 216–217

Q

Q fever pneumonia, 37
  radiography of, 37

R

Radiation injury, 177–180
  clinical course, 178–179
  pathology, 177–178
  radiographic course, 179–180
    acute changes, 179
    chronic changes, 179–180
Radiography
  chest
    of immunocompromised host, 53–56
    in intensive care unit (see under Intensive care unit)
    exposure difference between lung and mediastinum, 213
    lung cancer, 74–75
    mobile, 211–212
      exposure latitude, 211–212
      exposure times, 211
      kilovolt in, 211–212
      patient positioning for, 211
      radiographic contrast, 211–212
    pulmonary mass, solitary, 72
    of silicosis (see Silicosis, radiography of)
Radiology (see Radiography)
Radionuclide studies: in pulmonary hypertension, 95
Respiration/ventilation mode, 212–215
Respiratory distress in newborn
  chest wall causes, 21
  mediastinal causes, 19–21
  pulmonary causes, 3–18
Rheumatoid arthritis, 201–202
  secondary causes of infiltrative disease, 202
  radiography of, 202
Rib neoplasms, 59
Rupture: diaphragm, 176–177
Rye classification: of Hodgkin's disease, 66

S

Saber-sheath trachea, 124
Sarcoidosis, 196–198
  causing tracheal narrowing, 124

radiography of, 197–198
Scanning (*see* Imaging)
Scleroderma, 202–203
  radiography of, 202–203
Sclerosis, progressive systemic, 202–203
  radiography of, 202–203
Septic embolism, pulmonary, 118–119
  radiography of, 119
Serratia marcescens pneumonia, 29
  radiography of, 29
Shunt: left-to-right, excluded in pulmonary hypertension, 91
Silicosis, 152–153
  pathology, 152
  radiography of
    complicated silicosis, 153
    simple silicosis, 153
Smoke inhalation, 187
Splenectomy, 55
Staphylococcal pneumonia, 25
  radiography of, 25
Streptococcal pneumonia, 25–26
  radiography of, 26
Swan-Ganz catheter, 216

T

Tachypnea: transient, of newborn, 6
Takayasu's arteritis, 166
Thermal injury, 187–188
Thoracostomy tube, 217
Thorax (*see* Chest)
Thromboembolism, pulmonary, 105–120
  (*See also* Embolism, pulmonary)
  chronic, 116–119
  key concepts, 105
  proximal, 116–119
  pulmonary hypertension and, 92
Thrombosis: deep vein, imaging of, 109
TNM definitions
  metastases, distant, 81
  nodal involvement, 81
  primary tumor, 80–81
Tomography, computed
  in emphysema, 143
  in pulmonary hypertension, 95
Toxoplasma gondii, 53
  radiography in, 53
Trachea, 121–126
  dilatation in connective tissue disorders, 125
  dimensions, 121
  dynamics, fluoroscopic assessment, 126
  key concepts, 121
  morphology, radiographic assessment, 125–126
  narrowing, diffuse, 121–126
    amyloidosis causing, 124
    causes of, 122
    fungal infections causing, 121–123
    mediastinal fibrosis causing, idiopathic, 125
    polychondritis causing, relapsing, 123
    sarcoidosis causing, 124
    tracheopathia osteochondroplastica causing, 124
    tuberculosis causing, 123

Wegener's granulomatosis causing, 123
saber-sheath, 124
widening, diffuse, 125–126
  causes of, 122
  tracheobronchomegaly causing, 125
Tracheobronchial fracture, 174
Tracheobronchomegaly: causing tracheal widening, 125
Tracheoesophageal
  atresia, 11
  fistula, 12–13
Tracheopathia of osteochondroplastica: causing tracheal narrowing, 124
Tracheostomy tube, 216
Trauma (see Lung, injury)
Tube(s)
  endotracheal, 215–216
  feeding, 217
  seen in ICU, 215–217
  thoracostomy, 217
  tracheostomy, 216
Tuberculosis, 37–40
  endobronchial, 40
  pathogenesis, 38
  primary, radiography of, 38–39
  pulmonary
    bronchopleural fistula complicating, 39
    complications, 39–41
    empyema complicating, 39
    manifestations, 39–41
    radiography of, indications for, 40
  reactivation, radiography of, 39
  tracheal narrowing due to, 123
Tumors (see Neoplasms)

U

Ultrasound: in pulmonary hypertension, 95

V

Varicella (see Herpes varicella)
Vasculitic syndromes
  classification, 161–167
  distinct, 162–163
Vasculitis
  hypersensitivity, 165–166
  immune complex disease and, 167
  pulmonary, 158–168
    key concepts, 158–159
    pathogenetic mechanisms, 160
    pathologic definitions, 159–160
    radiologic-pathologic correlation in, 167–168
Vasoconstriction: in pulmonary hypertension, 89
Vein
  azygous, and pulmonary edema, 101
  deep vein thrombosis, imaging of, 109
  pulmonary vein pressure increase in pulmonary hypertension, 88
  pulmonary veno-occlusive disease and pulmonary hypertension, 92–93
Venography: lower limb, in pulmonary embolism, 108

Ventilation/perfusion scanning: of pulmonary embolism, 111–114
Ventilation/respiration mode, 212–215
Ventriculography: to exclude shunt and Eisenmenger's physiology in pulmonary hypertension, 91
Vessels
  loss in pulmonary hypertension, 89
  luminal, obstruction in pulmonary hypertension, 89
  pedicle
    landmarks of, 100
    pulmonary edema and, 101
  pulmonary vascular resistance, 87
    increase in pulmonary hypertension, 88
Virus(es)
  adenovirus causing pneumonia, 32–33
  cytomegalovirus causing pneumonia in immunocompromised hosts, 33
  disease, systemic, with pneumonia, 33
  Epstein-Barr, causing pneumonia, 33
  herpes (see Herpes)
  pneumonia due to (see Pneumonia, viral)
V/Q scan interpretation: in pulmonary embolism, 113

W

Water: extravascular lung, 218–219
Wegener's granulomatosis (see Granulomatosis, Wegener's)
Wilson-Mikity syndrome, 7

Z

Zoster (see Herpes varicella-zoster)